Classics in Psychiatry

TOTAL ABOLITION OF PERSONAL RESTRAINT IN THE TREATMENT OF THE INSANE

ROBERT GARDINER HILL

ARNO PRESS

A New York Times Company

New York · 1976

Editorial Supervision: EVE NELSON

————◆————

Reprint Edition 1976 by Arno Press Inc.

CLASSICS IN PSYCHIATRY
ISBN for complete set: 0-405-07410-7
See last pages of this volume for titles.

Manufactured in the United States of America

Publisher's Note: This book was reprinted
from the best available copy.

————◆————

Library of Congress Cataloging in Publication Data

Hill, Robert Gardiner, 1811-1878.
    Total abolition of personal restraint in the
treatment of the insane.

    (Classics in psychiatry)
    A lecture delivered at the Mechanics' Insti-
tution, Lincoln, Eng., June 21, 1838.
    Reprint of the 1839 ed. published by Simpkin,
Marshall, London.
    1. Psychiatry--Early works to 1900. 2. Psy-
chiatry hospital care. I. Title. II. [DNLM:
WM H646t 1839a]
    RC340.H65 1975   362.2'1   75-16725
    ISBN 0-405-07433-6

TOTAL ABOLITION OF PERSONAL RESTRAINT IN
THE TREATMENT OF THE INSANE.

A

LECTURE

ON

THE MANAGEMENT OF LUNATIC ASYLUMS,

AND THE

TREATMENT OF THE INSANE;

DELIVERED AT THE MECHANICS' INSTITUTION, LINCOLN,

ON THE 21st OF JUNE, 1838:

WITH

STATISTICAL TABLES,

ILLUSTRATIVE OF THE COMPLETE PRACTICABILITY OF THE SYSTEM
ADVOCATED IN THE LECTURE.

BY

ROBERT GARDINER HILL,

MEMBER OF THE ROYAL COLLEGE OF SURGEONS, LONDON;

HOUSE-SURGEON OF THE LINCOLN LUNATIC ASYLUM.

LONDON:
SIMPKIN, MARSHALL AND CO., STATIONERS HALL COURT,
AND S. HIGHLEY, 32, FLEET STREET,
LINCOLN: W. AND B. BROOKE.

LINCOLN:
W. AND B. BROOKE, PRINTERS, HIGH-STREET.

TO THE

RIGHT HONORABLE THE PRESIDENT,

THE VICE-PRESIDENTS AND GOVERNORS,

OF THE

LINCOLN LUNATIC ASYLUM,

THE FOLLOWING PAGES

ARE RESPECTFULLY INSCRIBED

BY THEIR GRATEFUL SERVANT,

THE AUTHOR.

PREFACE.

THE object of the following Lecture is simply to advocate the Total Abolition of Severity, of every species and degree, as applied to Patients in our Asylums for the Insane; and with this view to shew,—*First*, That such Abolition is in theory highly desirable, and *Secondly*, That it is practicable: in proof of which assertions the present state of the Lincoln Lunatic Asylum is adduced. There such a system is in actual and successful operation —the theory verified by the practice.* It

* The want of information upon this subject, even in respectable quarters, is much to be lamented, and is too well proved by extracts from the Glasgow and Nottingham Reports. Were the matter a theoretical question, such language as theirs might be used: but experience and facts cannot be evaded by mere words. Let our Glasgow and Nottingham neighbours honestly *make the attempt*, and they will succeed: and the necessity for "taking a month to tame a patient" (words lately addressed to me by an Attendant at the Glasgow Asylum in excuse for restraining a new patient) will disappear. Such matters should not be left to the discretion of the Attendants.

may be proper to state here, that the principle
of Mitigation of Restraint to the utmost extent
that was deemed consistent with safety, was
ever the principle pressed upon the attention
of the Boards of the Lincoln Asylum by its
humane and able Physician, Dr. Charlesworth:
at his suggestion many of the more cruel instru-

*Extract from the Twenty-fifth Annual Report of the Directors of the
Glasgow Royal Asylum for Lunatics.* 1839.

 " In connexion with other improvements in the treatment of the Insane,
" we, at an early period of our Institution, made it our especial study to render
" the means of coercion, when necessary, as gentle and as little irritating as
" possible ; but some degree of personal restraint is in many cases indispensable,
" and however gratifying the idea may be to the speculative philanthropist, the
" entire abolition of coercion is too often compensated by concealed severity.
" When we hear a vulgar and uneducated Keeper boasting that, by a glance of
" his eye, or the turn of his finger, he can control a whole ward of the Insane, we
" can guess pretty well how this seemingly mysterious power was acquired ; and
" it would be well if those who visit Mad-houses would carefully study the coun-
" tenances of the Lunatics when the Keeper approaches, and when he turns his
" back to the patient. An attentive observer might thus sometimes discover a
" strong and instructive contrast between the subdued and counterfeited expression
" in the one case, and the suspicious and revengeful scowl in the other."

*Extract from the Twenty-eighth Annual Report of the state of the General
Lunatic Asylum, near Nottingham.* 1838.

 " Without entertaining Utopian ideas, on the subject of the total abolition
" of all restraint in the treatment of Insanity, constant and unwearied attention
" has been directed to do as much without it as the welfare and safety of the
" Insane would admit."

ments of restraint were long since destroyed, very many valuable improvements and facilities gradually adopted, and machinery set in motion, which has led to the unhoped for result of actual Abolition, under a firm determination to work out the system to its utmost applicable limits.* To his steady support, under many difficulties, I owe chiefly the success which has attended my plans and labours. He originated the requisite alterations and adaptations in the Building, and threw every other facility in the way of accomplishing the object.

Experience has shewn that the mere partial mitigation of restraint is not in itself a safe system, suicides not having diminished under it†; if any conclusion may be drawn from the few cases, it would appear on the contrary that there is not any safety, when the Attendants are not compelled to rely wholly upon

* See proceedings of the Lincoln Lunatic Asylum relative to Classification, Inspection, and other matters bearing upon the subject of Restraint, in the Appendix (A.)

† See Table of Suicides, in the Appendix (D.)

Inspection. This propensity cannot be counter-
acted by any other means, than the constant
supervision of attendants by day, and a watch
by night, aided by the remission of ignorant
and cruel usages which no doubt have often
driven the insane sufferer to seek in suicide
the only means of escape. The disappearance
of suicide under the system of Total Abolition
has confirmed this opinion. By the annexed
Tables it will be seen, that not one fatal accident has occurred in this Asylum since the
Total Abolition of Restraints.

The Appendix (A,) abounds in curious and
instructive matter, which will be found eminently useful in other Institutions. It contains
the proceedings of the Boards and Officers for
a course of years in carrying out the great
principles of Construction, Classification, Public Inspection, Pervision, exoneration of the
Attendants from domestic duties, and other
matters which have directly or indirectly borne
upon the final extinction of restraint. These
memoranda are peculiarly valuable, as not
being merely wild and exaggerated views of

the moment, but matters of practice slowly, gradually, and perseveringly worked out from point to point, as experience and an indefatigable spirit of benevolence directed the course. The Author is proud to have learned in such a school, and gladly owns the obligation.

Lincoln Lunatic Asylum,
April 13, 1839.

CONTENTS.

———

LECTURE,

———

Mr. President,
    Ladies and Gentlemen,

       In addressing you this evening, I have at least two decided advantages :—In the first place, I need not enter into any lengthened exposition of my design,—I need not explain a mass of difficult and technical phrases, as a necessary preliminary to the right understanding of what I propose to lay before you. Happily my subject requires not such aid : it has *one* recommendation, and that one, I believe to be all-sufficient to win your favorable attention :—it asks nothing of you beyond the exercise of your own good sense and benevolent feelings, to make you understand and take an interest in its objects.

I plead the cause of a class of your fellow-creatures, too long alas! neglected, but surely a class demanding, if ever any did demand, the sympathy of every humane heart, and the compassion of every feeling bosom. Such a cause, however little it may derive from its advocate, will never be dismissed hence without an attentive hearing.—In the next place, I have not far to search for an example illustrative of the practice to which I shall this evening direct your attention. Turn your eyes to that noble Edifice, which is at once one of the greatest ornaments of modern date, which this City can boast, and a lasting memorial of your charity and benevolence. Thence are derived all my materials: there I have not only matured the plans, but have also witnessed and rejoiced in their complete success. There at this moment they are in full operation; and, I may be allowed to state, that they have already produced results beyond even my own most sanguine expectations. I do not ask your assent to my unsupported assertion of this: the Tables I have drawn up, and which I now hold in my hand, are a proof of it. Thence therefore I derive the illustrations of my theory;—practical results which may be seen and examined by any of you;—

examples of success which cannot be gain-
sayed—which cannot be controverted. It is
no visionary scheme ;—the proof is open to all
that I now address.

Counting, therefore upon a kind and favorable reception from you, I come at once to the
point, and ask whether, after having raised
such a noble edifice as the Lincoln Lunatic
Asylum for a class of beings, who have no
other hope of recovery on this side the grave,
it be not worth while to consult their personal
comfort and happiness, especially if that comfort and that happiness be found by experience
mainly conducive to their early restoration to
health and sanity, and consequently conducive
also in the highest degree to the charitable
objects for which the building was erected ?
I anticipate the answer of every one of you :
but readily as this is granted, conformable as
it is to the plain and obvious dictates of sense
and humanity, the history and experience of
past times will shew us that this principle has
not been acted upon in the case of the poor
Maniac—far from it. The inmates of a Lunatic
Asylum, (I speak not of our own in particular—
it's date being comparatively recent, just when
a more enlightened system had begun to dawn,
—but of every one without exception through-

out the whole continent of Europe,) were treated more like the savage and untameable beast of the forest than as human beings ; and the bare recital of their sufferings under this system of cruelty, is almost too horrible to be heard of or to be believed. The testimonies and facts which I shall bring forward will, however, shew that I have not overdrawn the picture.

Of the utility, however, of such Institutions, when conducted on humane principles, and when every effort, regardless of trouble or inconvenience, is concentrated towards one grand point—the benefit of the patient—there can be but one opinion. I shall not here dilate on the nature and causes of Insanity ; although this is a subject which would furnish matter well worthy the consideration, not only of professional men, but also of the philanthropist, the moralist, and even the divine. But it would lead me into a wider field than we have opportunity at present to range through and explore. My only wish, with reference to this part of my subject, is to furnish you with such information as may shew you the improbability, (I had almost said moral impossibility) of an insane person's regaining the use of his reason, except by removing him early to some Institution for that purpose. If such a result is ever attained without the adoption of this plan, it is either a very rare occurrence indeed, or it has ensued from change of residence, of scene, and of persons around, combined with a mode of treatment in some measure resembling that which can be fully adopted only in a Building constructed for the purpose.*

On the first attack of Insanity (from whatever cause arising) there is either some one all-engrossing idea haunting the brain like a

---

* " In an Asylum the patient is more carefully watched, and with less restraint than in a private house. What can be done with a furious individual in an apartment or in a house, however large it might be? For the sake of his own preservation, it would be necessary to tie him down to his bed, which would increase his delirium and fury, while in an Asylum he might indulge in his incoherence with less danger to himself and others. There, too, the management is better understood, the servants are more experienced, and the arrangement of the building allows the patient to be removed from one part to another according to his condition, the efforts which he makes, and his approach to reason."

" Their number (i. e. of the attendants) exhibits an amount of power which overcomes the most furious patient, and very frequently renders the employment of force unnecessary. A patient might be tempted to resist one or two ; but when he sees a body of four or five calm, powerful, and determined individuals, ready on the instant to execute the orders of the superintendent, the folly and fruitlessness of any resistance, becomes too apparent to allow him to make any effort."

" Example, which has such power over the determinations of men in general, exerts a great influence over the insane. We must bear in mind that the insane frequently exhibit great sagacity in judging of what passes around them. The cure and departure of one patient inspires others with confidence, the hope of recovery, and an assurance that they too will be liberated when cured."

" The care bestowed on them in the bosom of their own families makes no good impression on them, while the attention which they receive from strangers is appreciated from its being new, and their having no right to expect it."— *Edinburgh Medical and Surgical Journal, Jan.* 1, 1839, *pages* 152, 153 & 154.

spectre, and continually suggested so long as
the patient remains in the same place, and surrounded by the same persons;—or there is a
strong dislike conceived against the latter, or
some one or more of them;—or there is a
moping melancholy, with an inclination to
suicide, which is increased by a continuance
among the same objects;—or lastly, there is an
unmanageable violence, which vents itself on
every thing within its reach, and frequently
in attempting to destroy the lives of others:
and in all these cases, so long as the patient
remains at home, *the exciting causes are
continually present and active.* A change of
scene is therefore necessary—a change of attendants is necessary—a system of watchfulness
is necessary—and many other requisites are
necessary, which cannot be even attempted
except in an Asylum. A private dwelling is
ill adapted to the wants and requirements of
such an unfortunate being, as will appear from
the sequel of my address; nor is it consistent
with the safety of others, that he should be
allowed to roam at large. Means are therefore resorted to, which, however indispensible
under *such* circumstances, generally complete
the misery of the patient, who is thereby cut
off, perhaps for ever, from all hope of recovery.

And, even if a private dwelling did contain all that is requisite, still there is little probability that the patient could derive much benefit from the management of persons, who are neither acquainted with a proper system of treatment, nor, if they were, could they possibly adopt it, and at the same time attend to any other business or occupation whatsoever. *A Lunatic demands the whole time and attention of his Guardians.*—In last year's Report of the Lincoln Asylum the following passage occurs :— " It cannot be too widely made known that in a properly constructed and well-regulated Asylum, the Insane may be treated not only much more easily and effectually, but also *much more mildly* than at their own homes, where the unadapted arrangements of the Dwelling and Grounds, and the presence of Relatives and Dependants, oppose unceasing impediments to Recovery, and often produce an aggravation of the complaint by the restraint and close confinement which may become unavoidable under the circumstances."*—Indeed it is not to be expected that a patient should have any thing like the same prospect of recovery under improper, as under proper treatment. If it were possible that we could

* Report for 1837, page 5.

have a return of the number of persons recovering under private* treatment compared
with the whole number of Lunatics subjected to
such treatment, the truth of my observation
would be amply verified. Of this, however,
we have full proof, that the early removal
of patients to a Building where proper attendance and care can be had, is essential,
*the probability of recovery decreasing in pro-
portion to the length of time, which may have
elapsed between the period of the attack and
that of the removal.*† This fact, together with
the certain knowledge that a large proportion are yearly discharged recovered from such
Establishments, is sufficiently demonstrative
of their utility. "Drs. Munro, Burrows, and
Ellis, declare that they cure 90 out of every
100 cases. Such a result proves, so far as the
practice of these observers is concerned, that
Insanity, instead of being the most intractable,
is the most curable of all diseases. Observe,
however, that this declaration *applies only to
recent cases, which have not existed for more
than three months*, and which have been treated
under the most favorable circumstances ; as the

---

* By private treatment, I mean simply treatment at their homes, by their
own friends.

† See Table 52, Appendix E.

patients either belonged to the independent classes, or were inmates of one of the most deservedly popular Institutions in England."* But, even taking the average proportion of cures without reference to such favorable circumstances, (and this surely is the safest plan), it ranks very high. In the Lincoln Asylum the recoveries per 100 patients of every date, average 38.3 ;† while the deaths (including not only deaths from maniacal exhaustion, and from suicide, but also from old age, from diseases, in short from every natural cause to which Lunatics, as well as others, are equally liable) average only 19.5 † out of every 100. At Hanwell, which until very lately, was conducted by Sir William Ellis, the proportion of deaths is somewhat greater, viz., 50.4 ‡ out of every 100. Recoveries 18.8. ‡ It may be observed that Sedentary Employments are encouraged at Hanwell,

---

* Browne on Insanity and Asylums for the Insane, page 69.

† Farr on the Statistics of English Lunatic Asylums, pages 6 and 9.

From the opening of the Institution, April 26, 1820, to December 31, 1838.
Recoveries per cent. (Re-admitted cases included) ... 39.86
———————— (Re-admitted cases struck off) ... 48.30
Deaths per cent. (Re-admitted cases included)......... 16.50
———————— (Re-admitted cases struck off)......... 20.00

R. G. H.

‡ Farr on the Statistics of English Lunatic Asylums, pages 6 & 9.

which has not been the case at Lincoln. *

The efficacy and utility of Asylums being indisputably established, it may be asked, ' How is it to be accounted for that so strong a feeling should exist against them, and that so large a majority of patients should be unwilling to enter them ?' The question is natural, and the answer is easy. If Asylums were now what they formerly were, little indeed could be urged in their favor. " There are few subjects into which man can enquire," says an able Journalist, " from which he will turn with as much horror, as from an investigation into the manner in which insane persons were formerly treated. Lashings, it is recorded, constituted the common mode of treatment received by these unhappy creatures at the hands of their ascetical keepers. When Asylums became general, the case was very little amended. Lunatics were regarded rather in the light of wild beasts, than of human beings, and the mode of managing them corresponded with this brutal and unworthy notion. In fact,

* I am decidedly opposed to all Employment of Lunatics by which dangerous implements are put into their hands. It is even proverbial that
 *   *   *   *   " edged tools,
Should not be placed in the hands of fools."
More accidents have arisen from this cause, perhaps, than any other. Besides air and exercise are more suited to such patients, and better calculated to restore the mind to cheerfulness and sanity.

neither medical men, nor the public at large, had any hope of a cure of the insane. Their rooms or cells were uniformly loathsome from dirt; and in many places on the Continent, Lunatics were confined in cages, through the bars of which food and straw were thrust in to them, and where they were daily exhibited to visitors, who paid a certain sum to see them, as is done with wild beasts."

" This picture might be greatly extended, but enough has been said for our present purpose. And to what period, think you, does this description apply? It is scarcely 20 years since nearly every word of it might be said with truth of the receptacles of the insane in Britain! It was only at that period that a better spirit spread abroad on the subject of Insanity. Asylums began to be regarded as places for the cure, not for the living burial, of Lunatics."[*]

I have chosen to give this account in the words of another, that I might not be charged with giving an overdrawn picture; but in truth what has been said is but a mere sketch of their wrongs. Instances could be brought forward, confirmed by undeniable testimony, of brutality at which the mind recoils with

* Chambers' Edinburgh Journal, No. 307.

horror : but humanity will draw a veil over
the unsightly picture, and only express a
hope that the system, if not its tragic records,
will ere long be buried in oblivion.

Yet while we are compelled to confess that
such was the treatment adopted in cases of
Insanity, at no very distant period, can we
wonder that a feeling, and a very strong feeling too, should be frequently manifested by
the afflicted and their friends against entering
these retreats ? It is only surprising that so
much of this feeling has been overcome as
is actually the case. The only account that
can be given—the only pretext—the only
shadow of an excuse that can be alleged in
palliation is, that Insanity was deemed incurable, and the insane person a dangerous and
ferocious animal, who could never again be
approached with safety, nor recovered from
his savage and destructive habits. The moment this error was exploded, a brighter day
began to dawn upon the poor maniac. "Earlier
than 20 years ago, a reforming impulse had
been given to the subject in some European
countries; but the spirit of improvement was
tardy in its operation."* It is not my intention to trace fully its rise and progress; but

Chambers' (ubi supra).

I cannot avoid placing before you a sketch of the first practical attempt at rational and moral treatment; and a more affecting account is not, I think, to be met with in the annals of our race.

" Towards the end of 1792, Pinel, after having many times urged the government to allow him to unchain the maniacs of the Bicêtre, but in vain, went himself to the authorities, and with much earnestness and warmth, advocated the removal of this monstrous abuse— Couthon, a member of the commune, gave way to M. Pinel's arguments, and agreed to meet him at the Bicêtre. Couthon then interrogated those who were chained, but the abuse he received, and the confused sounds of cries, vociferations, and clanking of chains in the filthy and damp cells, made him recoil from Pinel's proposition. ' You may do what you will with them,' said he, ' but I fear you will become their victim.' Pinel instantly commenced his undertaking. There were about 50 whom he considered might without danger to the others be unchained, and he began by releasing twelve, with the sole precaution of having previously prepared the same number of strong waistcoats, with long sleeves, which could be tied behind the back, if necessary.

The first man on whom the experiment was to be tried was an English captain, whose history no one knew, as he had been in chains 40 years. He was thought to be one of the most furious among them; his keepers approached him with caution, as he had in a fit of fury killed one of them on the spot with a blow from his manacles. He was chained more rigorously than any of the others. Pinel entered his cell unattended, and calmly said to him, ' Captain, I will order your chains to be taken off, and give you liberty to walk in the court, if you will promise me to behave well and injure no one.' ' Yes, I promise you,' said the maniac; ' but you are laughing at me, you are all too much afraid of me.' ' I have six men' answered Pinel, ' ready to enforce my commands, if necessary. Believe me then on my word, I will give you your liberty if you will put on this waistcoat.'

" He submitted to this willingly, without a word: his chains were removed, and the keepers retired, leaving the door of the cell open. He raised himself many times from his seat, but fell again on it, for he had been in a sitting posture so long that he had lost the use of his legs; in a quarter of an hour he succeeded in maintaining his balance, and with tottering steps came to the door of his dark cell. His first look was at the sky, and he cried out enthusiastically, ' how beautiful!' During the rest of the day he was constantly in motion, walking up and down the staircases, and uttering short exclamations of delight. In the evening he returned of his own accord into his cell, where a better bed than he had been accustomed to had been prepared for him, and he slept tranquilly. During the two succeeding years which he spent in the Bicêtre, he had no return of his previous paroxysms, but even rendered himself useful by exercising a kind of authority over the insane patients, whom he ruled in his own fashion.

" The next unfortunate being whom Pinel visited was a soldier of the French Guards, whose only fault was drunkenness: when once he lost self command by drink he became quarrelsome and violent, and the more dangerous from his great bodily strength. From his frequent excesses, he had been discharged from his corps, and he had speedily dissipated his scanty means. Disgrace and misery so depressed him that he became insane : in his paroxysms he believed himself a general, and fought those who would not acknowledge his rank. After a furious struggle of this sort, he was brought to the Bicêtre in a state of the greatest excitement. He had now been chained for 10 years, and with greater care than the others, from his having frequently broken his chains with his hands only. Once when he broke loose, he defied all his keepers to enter his cell until they had each passed under his legs; and he compelled eight men to obey this strange command. Pinel, in his previous visits to him, regarded him as a man of original good nature, but under excitement, incessantly kept up by cruel treatment; and he had promised speedily to ameliorate his condition, which promise alone had made him more calm. Now he anounced to him that he should be chained no longer, 'and to prove that he had confidence in him, and believed him to be a man capable of better things, he called upon him to assist in releasing those others who had not reason like himself; and promised, if he conducted himself well, to take him into his own service.' The change was sudden and complete. No sooner was he liberated than he became obliging and attentive, following with his eye every motion of Pinel, and executing his orders with as much address as promptness: he spoke kindly and reasonably to the other patients, and during the rest of his life was entirely devoted to his deliverer. And 'I can never hear without emotion (says Pinel's son) the name of this man, who some years after this occurrence shared with me the games of my childhood, and to whom I shall feel always attached.'

" In the next cell were three Prussian soldiers, who had been in chains for many years, but on what account no one knew. They were in general calm and inoffensive, becoming animated only when conversing together in their own language, which was unintelligible to others. They were allowed the only consolation of which they appeared sensible,—to live together. The preparations taken to release them alarmed them, as they imagined the keepers were come to inflict new severities ; and they opposed them violently when removing their irons. When released they were not willing to leave their prison, and remained in their habitual posture. Either grief or loss of intellect had rendered them indifferent to liberty.

" Near them was seen an old priest, who was possessed with the idea that he was Christ : his appearance indicated the vanity of his belief ; he was grave and solemn ; his smile soft and at the same time severe, repelling all familiarity; his hair was long and hung on each side of his face, which was pale, intelligent and resigned. On his being once taunted with a question that ' if he was Christ he could break his chains,' he solemnly replied, ' Frustra tentaris Dominum tuum.' His whole life was a romance of religious excitement. He undertook on foot pilgrimages to Cologne and Rome; and made a voyage to America for the purpose of converting the Indians: his dominant idea became changed into actual mania, and on his return to France he announced himself as the Saviour. He was taken by the Police before the Archbishop of Paris, by whose orders he was confined in the Bicêtre as either impious or insane. His hands and feet were loaded with heavy chains, and during twelve years he bore with exemplary patience this martyrdom and constant sarcasms. Pinel did not attempt to reason with him, but ordered him to be unchained in silence, directing at the same time that every one should imitate the old man's reserve, and never speak to him. This order was rigorously observed, and produced on the patient a more decided effect than either chains or a dungeon; he became humiliated by this unusual isolation, and after hesitating for a long time, gradually introduced himself to the society of the other patients. From this time his notions became more just and sensible, and in less than a year he acknowledged the absurdity of his previous prepossession, and was dismissed from the Bicêtre.

"In the course of a few days, Pinel released fifty-three maniacs from their chains : among them were men of all conditions and countries ; workmen, merchants, soldiers, lawyers, &c. The result was beyond his hopes. Tranquillity and harmony succeeded to tumult and disorder, and the whole discipline was marked with a regularity and kindness which had the most favorable effect on the insane themselves ; rendering even the most furious more tractable." *

Previous to this trial, moral and humane treatment was never attempted. " The mind was left to recover its native strength and buoyancy spontaneously." † " Classification was never thought of : criminals, lunatics, the furious and the gentle, were compelled to live promiscuously."‡ Instruments of restraint of the most cruel description were constantly

* The British and Foreign Medical Review, No. 1, page 286.
† Browne on Insanity and Asylums for the Insane, page 223.   ‡ Ibid.

resorted to ; instruments which deprived the patient of all power and command over himself, and reduced him at once to the most abject state of helplessness, misery, filth, and wretchedness. Food was thrust down the throat, and the mouth forced open by one of those instruments of cruelty, the use of which was occasionally attended with fatal results. 'The wretched victims of this barbarous system were left to wallow in their filth on heaps of straw—no fires allowed—their extremities sometimes in a state of mortification through excessive cold—and not even the sexes separated from each other.

I turn with pleasure from this picture to the more humane and enlightened system, which followed the attempt of the intelligent and immortal Pinel, and in which the Quakers took the lead in this country in their admirable Institution the Retreat. To the credit of all concerned, it may be truly asserted, that when once it was proved that moral means were efficacious, improvement rapidly advanced. Every where the light seemed to flash upon mankind, that these unfortunate beings were still of the same race and order with themselves, and had some claim to an attempt at least at kind and feeling treatment. The attempt once made, its efficacy was undeniable; and now there does not exist an Institution where *kindness* is not held forth as the principal means resorted to for the recovery of the insane. The very name of "*Mad-house*" is almost forgotten. In place thereof an "*Asylum*" is offered for these poor creatures:—a place of refuge, of shelter from injury, of comfortable retreat, until the storm be overpast:—a place where every want is attended to, every reasonable wish gratified. Still, however, much remains to be done: and it is mainly with the view of stating what may yet be accomplished, and not merely stating, but proving that statement by incontestible examples, that I now address you. *I wish to complete that which Pinel began.* I assert then in plain and distinct terms, *that in a properly constructed building, with a sufficient number of suitable attendants, restraint is never necessary, never justifiable, and always injurious, in all cases of Lunacy whatever.* I assert the possibility of the total banishment of instruments of restraint, and all other cruelties whatsoever. I assert that the Asylum of your own City, when completed, may be conducted without a single instance of restraint occurring from one year's end to another. I trust I may here calculate upon your indulgence when I venture to read an extract or two from the Reports of our Asylum for 1837 and 1838, although they have reference to myself, and my opinions.

(1837). " The present House-Surgeon has expressed his own belief, founded on experience in this house, that it may be possible to conduct an Institution for the Insane without having recourse to the employment of any Instruments of Restraint whatsoever. He has certainly made a striking advance towards verifying this opinion, by conducting the Male (the completed) side of the house, with but a solitary* instance of such restraint, either by day or by night, during the course of the sixteen last months, and that applied only for about six hours, during his absence; nor is it impossible, when the Buildings can be finished, that an example may be offered of an Asylum, in which undivided personal attention towards the Patients shall be altogether substituted for the use of Instruments.

" By the degree of approach to this Result

---

* This is an error, there was another instance amounting to eight hours. This occurred in consequence of a bench ordered many months before not having been fixed in the floor, in place of loose forms applicable as instruments of offence by the Patients.

of sound Construction, of Management, **and**
of Official Conduct, ought the excellence **of**
every Public Asylum to be tested."*

(1838). " There is now an increased confidence that the anticipations of the last year
may be fulfilled, and that '.An example may
' be offered of a Public Asylum, in which undi-
' vided personal attention towards the Patients
' shall be altogether substituted for the use of
' Instruments of restraint.' The bold conception of pushing the mitigation of restraint to the
extent of actually and formally abolishing the
practice, mentioned in the last Report as due
to Mr. Hill the House-Surgeon, seems to be
justified by the following abstract of a statistical Table, showing the rapid advance of the
abatement of restraints in this Asylum, under
an improved Construction of the Building,
Night-watching, and attentive Supervision.
We may venture to affirm, that this is the first
frank Statement of the common practice of restraints, hitherto laid before a British Public."†
(See Table in the Appendix C.)

Suffer me now to bring forward a few examples illustrative of the efficacy of proper
treatment without restraint; premising that
the very restoration to liberty of Patients

---

* Report for 1837, page 5.   † Report for 1838, page 4.

brought to us under all manner of restraints, and apparently ungovernably furious, has often an immediate good effect in restoring them to repose, and in one or two instances, almost to sanity. Indeed the violence is much oftener the result of coercion than of the malady.

Nos. 547, 549, and 551 :—These Patients were admitted in January, 1836. They had all been confined in a workhouse for a number of years—say between fifteen and twenty. During this period of time they scarcely knew what it was to be at liberty; I have understood that they were chained both day and night to their bedsteads, and kept in a state so filthy that it was heart sickening to go near them. They were usually restrained with the strait-waist-coat, with collars round their necks ;—the collars being fastened with chains or straps to the upper portions of their bedsteads, to pre-vent them (as I have since been informed) from biting their bed-clothes: their feet were chained to the bedsteads with iron leg-locks, to which chains were attached. One of the poor crea-tures, who no doubt had her lower extremities at liberty, was so deformed from the continued confinement, that she was unable to move about; her limbs having become contracted to such a degree that her feet were drawn up until the soles were even with the lower part of her back : when moved from one room to another it was necessary for an attendant to carry her. These individuals *have never been personally restrained since their admission :* one of them I once placed under seclusion for a few hours only; but beyond that, no coercive means whatever have been employed. Two of these patients have been restored to habits of cleanliness :—one in particular now spends the greater part of her time in knitting, sewing, &c. Of course they have not been so orderly in their conduct as many of their companions; but is this to be wondered at, when for such a number of years they had been treated more like brutes than human beings? The crippled patient died a few months since of Consumption.

1838, April 12.—No. 662, æt. 20.—This patient has been readmitted this afternoon. She was brought in a strait-waistcoat, in a state of the greatest excitement. Five persons could scarcely bring her. She is single, and a member of the Baptist persuasion. This attack came on about a week since; the former about three years ago, from which she recovered after remaining in this Establishment about three or four months. She raves chiefly on religious topics, and is subject to sudden and violent fits of phrenzy. During the former attack she attempted self-destruction by jumping into a stone pit; she occasionally destroys her wearing apparel. Grief and religious excitement are assigned as the immediate exciting causes of the attack. 8. P M.—She has been very active in her personal exertions, and is unable to control herself.

April 13.—She has been under watch, and has been restless the whole of the night; she is still very active in her personal exertions, but more tractable than she was yesterday.

April 14.—She has become quiet and orderly.

April 15.—She continues calm and well behaved.

April 18.—The patient who was brought here on the 12th instant, confined with a strait-waistcoat, and guarded by several attendants, is already so far recovered as to have lost all disposition towards any inordinate action, and has been removed this morning to the Moderate Patients' Gallery. It cannot be doubted, indeed she has herself stated, that *the irritation of personal restraint had occasioned the excitement she at first exhibited.* The strait-waistcoat was instantly taken off on her admission.

April 20.—She has been removed to the Convalescent Patients' Apartment, and is now employed in needle-work.

From April 20 to June 11 inclusive.—Employed in household-work, needle-work, &c., &c.

June 11.—She has been discharged this day by the Weekly Board of Governors. When discharged she applied for the situation of kitchen maid, and was engaged.

1838, April 5.—No. 661, æt. 52.—This man has been received this morning. He is a labourer, married—with a family of six children. He has attended the Church regularly, and has also for many years attended the Wesleyan meetings. The first attack of Insanity he experienced was in his 29th year, when he was confined for thirteen weeks in Mr. ——'s Establishment at ——, where he recovered. This his second attack exhibited itself about ten days since, and no cause can be assigned for it except some recent religious excitement. He is subject to sudden fits of phrenzy, in one of which he escaped from his friends in a state of nudity;—he has conceived a strong dislike to the persons who have taken an active part in restraining him. He has neither attempted to injure himself, nor any other person. He has been confined in a strait-waistcoat since the commencement of the attack. Three men accompanied him hither. 8 p. m.—Since his admission he has been rolling about the floor of the Refractory Patients' Gallery : he has also been jumping and running to and fro';—he has just run violently against the gallery door, and broken it.

April 6.—He is very restless and incoherent, and has been so the whole of the night; —he is again rolling on the floor of the gallery, —I have desired the attendant not to leave him, for fear he should get hurt by any of the other patients.

April 7.—Though not so active in his personal exertions he is still restless,—complains of thirst ;—I have ordered the attendant to offer him cold water frequently during the day and night. He has slept under watch since his admission.

April 10.—He is not so restless, and is certainly improved in health.

April 14.—He continues to improve.

April 18.—He has lost all disposition to any inordinate action, and has this morning been removed to the Moderate Patients' Gallery.

April 21.—He is rational, quiet, and well behaved.

April 28.—He has been employed in household work and in gardening, since the 18th instant.

From April 29 to June 11 inclusive.—Has been employed in the wash-house;—has occasionally been allowed to go into the town accompanied by an attendant.

June 11.—Has been discharged this day. (Recovered.)

1838, April 23.—No. 664, æt. 28.—This patient has been received this morning. He is married, is a labourer, and a member of the Methodist persuasion. He has always been considered a sober, industrious, and respectable person. This his first attack came on a few weeks since, previous to which for a fortnight or three weeks he was observed to be more than usually devout and enthusiastic in his religious exercises. He is subject to sudden fits of phrenzy, but his certificate does not state whether he is dangerous or otherwise. Religious excitement is assigned as the immediate exciting cause of his Insanity. It appears the malady has been much aggravated by the use of the strait-waistcoat and other instruments of restraint. The persons accompanying him informed me, that he had been bound down to his bedstead for the three or four last weeks, and

that his health was much injured in consequence. His appearance is indeed ghastly, and
owing to his long confinement he has not the
proper use of his lower extremities. He has
also large sores upon his back. 7 P. M.—He
has been very quiet since his admission, but is
now restless, talkative, and noisy.

April 24.—He has been under watch;—
has passed a restless night;—is somewhat noisy
this morning, and talks much on religious subjects, fancying that he has converted to his own
views the workmen employed at the—Union.

April 25.—He is now tractable.

April 26.—He is improving.

April 30.—He is quiet and orderly, and
has been removed to the Moderate Patients'
Gallery.

May 1.—He is rational, calm, and well
behaved, and has been removed to the Convalescent Patients' Apartment. He is gaining
strength rapidly, and recovering the proper
use of his lower extremities.

From May 1 to May 25 inclusive.—Improving in health.

May 26.—He has recovered his health.
He has been permitted this day to go beyond
the walls, accompanied by an attendant and
one of the other patients.

From May 26 to June 11 inclusive.—Employed in the garden, yards, &c.

June 11.—He has been discharged this day. (Recovered).

This man must have died had the restraint been continued, so much had his health suffered from the impossibility of attending to himself, and to his natural wants.

No. 449.—Farmer. Married man. This furious patient was admitted on the 9th of January, 1834, aged 50. The malady in this case is hereditary, affording a lamentable exemplification of that law of nature—the impress of Nature's God—by which parents transmit to their offspring not merely the outward resemblance of feature, nor the yet more striking individual peculiarities of gait, manner, and action, so often observed to descend in this way ;* but also the physical conformation and constitution of those exquisitely formed internal organs, so intimately connected with the nobler powers of man—the mind and its energies and operations. Mania, then, being in some instances hereditary, it is clear that in

* Thus far the observation holds good throughout almost the whole animal kingdom, except in cases of transformations, as of the caterpillar to the butterfly; and it forms that bond of similarity in the same species amid the interminable variety of the individuals that compose it, which is one of the great charms of animated nature.

those instances it must depend on some organic conformation or constitution, which is transmitted from sire to son ; and from the accurate investigations and experiments made of late years, little doubt remains that the brain is the organ in question. *How*, indeed, a certain conformation of brain is connected with certain mental capacities or mental delusions, or how certain modes of life and conduct conduce to bring about that state of brain in those hereditarily predisposed to it, and even in others not so inheriting that predisposition, remains a subject of curious and not unprofitable speculation. But to return to my narrative. His malady first shewed itself in January, 1831. He had then been long given to habits of intoxication, indulging freely in the use of ale and ardent spirits. Foreseeing clearly the effect of these habits, as respected his fortune and means of livelihood, he had a terrible dread of impending poverty; and so horribly did this prospect haunt his imagination, that unable to discontinue those pernicious habits, the dire effects of which he so keenly and remorsefully anticipated, he attempted self-destruction by knocking his head violently against a wall. He was, however, discharged on trial on the 24th of October, 1834, having been an inmate of the Asylum nine months and a fortnight. Until the month of June following no symptoms of his former malady appeared, and in that interval he managed his affairs with considerable discretion, and conducted himself with decency, industry, and sobriety. But about the period mentioned he again indulged, as before, in the too free use of fermented liquors, and the consequence was a recurrence of his malady, and he was once more remanded to the Asylum. His friends stated that he had become quite violent and unmanageable, that he had attempted to destroy his wife with a garden fork which he had latterly kept in his bed-room, together with a gun and other formidable weapons. They further stated that he had broken some windows at the Rectory of the village where he resided, and that his conduct and demeanour towards several of his neighbours had been violent in the extreme. At the time of my appointment to the Asylum, he was suffering extremely from depression of spirits: he would often weep bitterly, supposing that his soul was for ever lost, and that he was *doomed* to suffer in hell fire. In the month of August, (1835), so bent did he appear on self-destruction, that I deemed it necessary to confine him to his bedstead for four successive nights; since which time, although frequently under the influence of violent paroxysms of phrenzy, he has not been personally restrained at all, the Dormitory and Night-watch (both of which were incipiently brought into operation within a week of the period named) having superseded the use of manacles at night. In May, 1836, being suddenly seized with one of his most outrageous paroxysms, he broke several panes of glass in the Moderate Patients' Apartment, where he had previously to that time conducted himself in a quiet and well behaved way. In doing this, he cut both his hands and wrists, and wounded one or two blood vessels: his wounds having been dressed he was removed without loss of time to the Refractory Patients' Gallery, where he has remained ever since in a state of great mental excitement, occasionally uttering the most profane and impious expressions, blaspheming God, throwing himself into attitudes of defiance, and threatening all around him with immediate and dire revenge. During these paroxysms he is watched most closely by the attendants, who however do not attempt to interfere with him, having found by long experience that even a word in remonstrance is but adding fuel to the fire. He is loud and vociferous, and will stand for hours together shouting to the walls, to the trees, and to the sky, believing that while so engaged he is building castles, palaces, and churches. He was employed for a length of time in his lucid intervals, in gardening, trenching, removing soil, &c., but so uncertain was his conduct and demeanour that it was ultimately considered necessary to keep him altogether unemployed, and to watch him closely. Yet even with this man, no coercive means are used—a proof at once that they may so far be dispensed with. He is believed to be of a cowardly disposition, and is so considered by the attendants. In one of his lucid intervals he informed me that when breaking the windows here, he made no doubt he was at his own village " playing away at the Rectory windows as on a former occasion :" and at the same time he expressed his contrition for having committed such an error. This individual is of athletic form, stands about six feet two inches high, and is of a morose and savage temper, although exhibiting frequently such strong marks of cowardice—but cruelty and cowardice are often strangely blended;—from his youth upwards he has ever been hasty, irritable, and vindictive.*

I beg leave now to read a letter from a patient to her friends:—

" Lincoln, January 4, 1837.

" Mrs. ——,

"When I was at —— I heard them say I was to come to Lincoln Lunatic Asylum, when I was quite feared seeing the severe confinements;—but this is quite different:—I am in the wards up and down where there are thirty-three female patients. I have not seen a strait-waistcoat, nor yet leather-sleeves, nor leg-locks, nor muzzles,† or other sorts of confinements;—say or do what you will there is no fault found;—the nurses all seem very loving and dutiful to the patients. If your finger only aches the House-Surgeon attends several times a day; and at night if he see any of them unruly he orders a nurse to sit up with them. The bed-rooms are carpeted, (feather beds most of them with hangings), wash-stands, basins, towels, looking glass, comb, and brush, and a nurse to attend us. We have tea twice a day, and as much toast

* This case was not read for fear of extending the lecture to too great a length. It was written a considerable time previous to the lecture, but as the case is a strong one I have thought proper to insert it.

† Muzzles and even gags have been employed in some Institutions to stifle the noise made by the more violent patients.

as we can eat;—milk and bread for our supper,
meat dinners every day, and different sorts of
puddings: the Matron of the Asylum stands
at the table, and asks whether we are all satisfied; and if any one wants more she orders
a nurse to bring it:—she wishes to see us all
comfortable. We go to bed at eight o'clock;
—we have nothing to do only to walk in the
gardens twice a day, and cards to play, and
other sorts of exercise. I never was better off
since I left my parents."

This proves that the system adopted is
gratifying to the patients, and thereby con-
duces to the comfort and healing of their
minds:—it will be necessary to add, that the
above patient had been confined in other Institutions for persons in her unfortunate situation.

But, it may be demanded, 'What mode of
treatment do you adopt, in place of restraint?
How do you guard against accidents? How
do you provide for the safety of the attendants?' In short, what is the substitute for
coercion? The answer may be summed up
in a few words, viz.—*classification*—*watchfulness*—*vigilant and unceasing attendance by
day and by night*—*kindness, occupation, and
attention to health, cleanliness, and comfort,*

and the total absence of every description of other occupation of the attendants. This treatment, in a properly constructed and suitable building, with a sufficient number of strong and active attendants always at their post, is best calculated to restore the patient; and all instruments of coercion and torture are rendered absolutely and in every case unnecessary.

In order, however, that this plan may be undeviatingly pursued, several essential requisites must unite :—

1. A suitable building must be provided, in an airy and open situation, with ground sufficient for several court-yards, gardens, and pleasure-grounds, commanding (if possible) a pleasing and extensive prospect.

2. There must be a proper classification of the patients, more *especially by night.**

3. There must be also a sufficient number of strong, tall, and active attendants, whose remuneration must be such as to secure persons of good character, and steady principle, to undertake their arduous duties. And

4. The House-Surgeon must exercise an

---

* Suicide under this system must be obviated by the constant attention of the House-Surgeon to the proper Classification of the Patients *by night.* Those disposed to suicide should always be placed in an Open Dormitory under watch. *Nothing else can prevent Suicide under any system whatever.*

unremitting control and inspection, in order that the plan may never, under any circumstances whatever, be deviated from in the slightest degree.

1 & 2. The nature of the Building required will be best understood from a view of the Classification, which renders a proper number of Apartments, Dormitories, Galleries, and Court-yards, unavoidably necessary. The following is a view of the Classification adopted in our Asylum.

Degrees of Rank—Three,—according to the payments made ; — viz., *First*, *Second*, *Third*.

Classes of Insanity—Three ;—viz., *Convalescent and Orderly, Moderate, Disorderly*.

The Day apartments consist of fourteen sitting-rooms, six galleries, and six dining-rooms.

The Convalescent and Orderly, and the Moderate of the first Rank have front rooms in the centre part of the House.

The Convalescent and Orderly of the second and third Ranks have front rooms at the extremities of the east and west Wings.

The Moderate Patients of the second and third Ranks have the use of Galleries and Sitting-rooms in the front, on the ground and

first floors;—these Galleries and Sitting-rooms
have a southern aspect.

The Disorderly of the Three Ranks have
the use of Galleries and Sitting-rooms which
project northward from the back of the Wings,
and have eastern and western aspects respectively.

The patients of the Three Ranks have at
all times access to the Courts, and the Convalescent and Orderly, and the Moderate are
allowed for many hours during the day to take
exercise on the lawn in front of the Establishment. As an indulgence, the quieter patients
are allowed occasionally to accompany the
porter and attendants into the town;—i. e. one
or two at a time:—occasionally as many as
six females have gone out together into the
fields.

The night apartments consist of two Open
Galleries or Dormitories, containing eighteen
beds each;—two Watch-rooms adjoining the
Dormitories, with eight beds each;—also four
rooms, with two beds each;—four rooms, with
three beds each;—and forty-eight rooms, with
one bed each:—besides the above there are
two Infirmaries for the first and second Rank
Patients, each containing three beds.

The long Dormitories are used for the

patients disposed to self-destruction :—the beds
in the Watch-rooms to those who destroy bed-
clothing,* and to the epileptics ;—the rooms

* I cannot forbear giving a case of this description, one of the worst which
has come under my observation ; in which, nevertheless, the necessity for restraint
was obviated by management.

1838, January 19.—No. 648, æt. 50.—This woman has been received to
day. She has two children. The attack commenced about seven months since:
she raves indifferently on various topics; is subject to sudden and violent fits of
phrenzy, and is very prone to destroy property. The immediate exciting cause
was the loss of her husband, who died insane. The patient attended upon
him during his illness, and up to his death, when she herself became insane.
She is very violent, and has been confined in a strait-waistcoat since the commencement of the attack. She is insensible to the ordinary calls of nature.

January 20.—She has passed a restless night. Her blankets were enclosed
in a strong case. She is very active in her personal exertions, and is noisy and
unruly.

January 22.—She is very refractory and quarrelsome.

January 25.—She is noisy and refractory.

January 26.—She continues noisy and refractory.

January 27.—She continues inattentive to the ordinary calls of nature. She
has destroyed her pillow-case and night-gown. Her blankets are enclosed in a
strong case.

January 29.—She tears her clothes, and commits other acts of gross ex-
travagance. A strong dress has been purchased for her.

January 30.—She continues to indulge her destructive propensity. I have
desired a nurse to sit by her in the day time.

February 9.—She has by some means effected an opening into her blanket-
case, and destroyed its contents to the amount of four blankets. I have ordered
that the pieces be collected, and quilted within the case.

February 10.—Much quieter during the night than she has been for some
time past. The nurse is obliged to remain with her in the day time, or else she
would not only destroy her own clothes, but those belonging to the other patients also.

February 11.—She has been very restless during the night. I have desired
the attendant on watch to visit her occasionally, which can be done without
neglecting the other patients, by having another nurse to sleep in the watch
room, and both to watch alternately.

February 25.—She is very violent and abusive.

March 8.—She is very incoherent and disorderly.

containing two and three beds each, to the
harmless and convalescent, and the single
bedded rooms to the harmless, the noisy, the
violent, or the insensible.*

April 9.—She still continues inattentive to the ordinary calls of nature, and
shews a strong inclination to destroy property.

April 19.—Having contrived several times of late to destroy her blanket-
case, a new case has been provided expressly for her: through this she has
made a hole with her teeth of the size of a crown piece, and has withdrawn the
whole of the woollen rags which the case contained. I have therefore ordered
that she be removed to the Watch-room, and every natural want regularly and
strictly attended to. The result is she has been quiet during the whole of the
night, as well as attentive to the requirements of nature.

April 20.—She has been under watch during the night, and I am happy to
say has not forfeited herself as regards either her propensity to destroy clothing,
or her inattention to the ordinary calls of nature. This individual had been
confined in a strait-waistcoat for many months previous to her admission here.

April 26.—She continues attentive to the ordinary calls of nature, being
under watch. She has certainly the power to control herself, and has latterly
endeavoured to do so in the day time as well as during the night. Previous to
her removal to the watch-room, she was told that if she would be cleanly in her
habits, she should be treated like the other patients; that is, instead of having
straw to sleep upon, she should have a flock bed. She promised to be clean,
and she has certainly kept her word up to the present period.

May 1.—She continues true to her word; and in the day time, though she
is very incoherent and mischievous, yet she is far more orderly than she used
to be.

May 7.—Clean and orderly.

1839, February 14.—She has continued so ever since. Had this patient
been put under restraint, she might have continued for ever a loathsome object,
insensible to every natural call: for the case was and is incurable.

* Recent observation has convinced me that if Dormitories could be provided for the Insensible patients also (those, I mean, who do not attend to the
calls of nature), *with Night-watches*, such might speedily be restored to habits of
cleanliness. This plan has been attended with the happiest effect in some late
instances: and indeed we have now few patients who are dirty in the day time,
why then in the night? Simply because they can be attended to only in the
day time, and if this attendance could be given also in the night, cleanliness
and self control would speedily supervene.

The greatest attention to personal cleanliness is observed. The patients have the use of the warm bath on admission : afterwards once in three weeks, and oftener if necessary : their feet are washed and their heads dry cleaned once a week, and their hands and faces daily :—their body-linen is changed twice a week ;—their bed-linen once in three weeks.

They have always water accessible in the galleries and sitting-rooms, so that it is scarcely possible for them to suffer from thirst.

The house is well ventilated ;—the bedroom windows are thrown open immediately after rising, and kept open throughout the day. The gallery and sitting-room windows are opened at meals and when they are taking exercise. They are also kept open during the whole of the night. The beds are thrown open, and not made up until breakfast is over.

It may be proper to add, that the apartments are now warmed by open fires,* by which any unwholesome tendency, (as well as the expense), of heated air-flues, is avoided. The introduction of sash doors is another excellent feature of this Institution ; for which,

---

* The fire places, however, are protected by a strong iron guard, lined with fine wire-work, which prevents the introduction of a stick or other combustible by the patients.

with his other valuable improvements, too great thanks cannot be given to Dr. Charlesworth, our senior physician. Some expedient is still required for the separation of the noisy from the quiet at night. I have long seen the necessity of this at Lincoln : these individuals must do considerable mischief to the others, and impede their return to a state of sanity.

3. A sufficient number of tall, strong, and active attendants, is absolutely necessary. The system of watchfulness is one which cannot be dispensed with. They must not be employed in any other way—their whole time and attention must be occupied with their charge. They must not be frequently changed —a change should never be made without actual necessity. They must be well remunerated, in order to secure persons of character and of trust. They must not speak angrily to the patients ; nevertheless they must be firm and determined in their demeanour towards them. An attendant ought on no occasion to have more than twelve or fifteen patients under his care. The same number of violent patients will require at least two to observe them. The laws of France assign one keeper to every ten patients.

Neither the patients nor attendants should be supplied with fermented liquors : such allowances have been found to engender strifes and contests amongst the former, and with the latter habits of intemperance, materially affecting the good order of the Establishment. In special cases where stimulants may be required, the faculty have power to order them.

In the treatment of the insane, medicine is of little avail,* except (of course) when they are suffering also from other diseases, to which lunatics as well as sane persons are liable. *Moral treatment with a view to induce habits of self-control, is all and every thing.* I have spoken of classification and watchfulness : but these things are done by their guardians, and have little or no reference to their feelings ; for they should if possible be watched without leading them to suppose that they are suspected of any thing improper or injurious.†

But occupation and kindness have especial

The use of the lancet, leeches, cupping-glasses, blisters, drastic purgatives, and the practice of shaving the head are totally proscribed in this Asylum as at Gloucester. The patients' bowels are kept open, their general health is attended to, and they are allowed a generous diet but no fermented liquor. The daily allowance of meat, bread, milk, &c., will be seen on reference to the Diet Table which is appended to this lecture.

† It is essential, however, that the patient should be aware that he is *observed* though not *suspected of wrong :* and aware also that the person who observes him is powerful enough to control him.

reference to the patient; and their object is
(as I have stated) to induce habits of self-control and cleanliness, which qualities are both
essential to recovery, and yet cannot possibly
be attained unto by a patient under restraint.
Out-door employments with moderate exercise
—cheerful society—the occasional presence of
friends and even of visitors—healthy recreations and amusements—the enjoyment of the
sweet music of spring, of a calm summer
evening—the care of a garden, or a shrubbery,
or the cultivation of rare and choice flowers—
all unite in producing a healthy tone, and
giving nerve and vigour to the shattered mind.
No patient should be *compelled* to work in
any way; but many of them, both males and
females, will voluntarily make themselves useful and be industrious; and in many cases their
services are very valuable. Sedentary employments are not good. The offices of religion
have a soothing and favorable effect on many :
—I have found the use of evening service, and
the calm and sober strain of piety which per-
vades the Liturgy, to be well adapted to these
unfortunate beings. Religious excitement of
the feelings is always bad, and has brought
a great number of patients to this, as well
as to every other Asylum. A patient should

never be terrified. " Fear is known, by those who have studied the feelings under which self-destruction is attempted, to be one of its most frequent causes. Strange to say, the apprehension of death itself leads to this act. ' It would seem,' says Dr. Reid, ' as if they rushed into the arms of death in order to shield themselves from the terror of his countenance.' "* Their feelings should be consulted as far as possible :—the bath of surprise, the rotatory chair, and all such devices cannot have a good effect.

Undivided personal attention towards the patients is now altogether substituted in this Establishment for the use of Instruments. During the last year there were but three instances of Restraint, and those amongst the females ; arising entirely from the unfinished and crowded state of the House, as did the two on the male side during the preceding year. When appointed House-Surgeon I confess I was but inexperienced ; for on finding patients under restraint I kept them so, merely because the attendants wished me so to do. Had their wishes alone been consulted, no doubt such treatment would have continued to the present time ;—but I soon observed

* Browne on Insanity and Asylums for the Insane, page 29.

that the wish on their part was a mere pretext for idleness, and a short time subsequent to this, I refused altogether to comply with their requests. Matters went on pretty well for three months; when the calls for restraint appeared so urgent, that I was induced to give way, and again the inmates were treated on the old principle. This was kept up for a few weeks, during which time I bestowed much attention on the patients, and observed frequently and assiduously the conduct of the attendants towards them. At length I felt convinced there was little occasion for the restraint, and resolved within myself to discontinue its use altogether. With this determination, I set at liberty those that were actually coerced; and from that time to the present, have had no occasion to resort to such measures, except in a few instances which arose, as I have before stated, from the unfinished and too crowded state of the Establishment. For a while after this I was frequently applied to for Restraint, but on each occasion I have refused it on the ground that it was unnecessary, having first visited the patient, and enquired into the circumstances. Thus it appears, that unless a Superintendent himself actually inspects the whole, and sees that his directions are accurately observed, he may be imposed upon, and the patients exposed to unnecessary severity.

Wherever Restraint may become necessary, *owing to the imperfect adaptation of the Building, or to a want of sufficient attendants,* the most simple means should be selected. On such an occasion, I do not know of any constraint which would be preferable to that of seclusion in a darkened room. In this Asylum when a patient misconducts himself, he is immediately removed to the Refractory Patients' Gallery, where he remains until he has pledged himself that his future conduct shall be more orderly. This is the only method I employ to induce habits of self-control. *A maniac is seldom known to break his word.*

Violent cases would be extremely rare in all Asylums, if the no-restraint system were generally adopted : as would Suicides also, if, in conjunction with the above, Dormitories and Night-watches were established ; but to dispense with Restraint altogether such must be the case, or the attempt would be attended with extreme danger. Without the Dormitories and Night-watches it would be necessary to restrain such as exhibited a tendency to suicide. Under this system, i. e. the no-restraint system, cases of insensibility to natural

H

calls would be seldom met with : to ensure the non-existence of such cases, the individuals must be removed from their own homes on the first appearance of the malady, or as soon afterwards as is practicable ; before such habits have been induced by the use of the strait-waistcoat or other instruments which confine the fingers, and thus disable the patient from assisting himself on natural occasions.

I forgot to mention, when speaking of the Watch-room, that we have a Clock fixed in this room which shews each time that the Watchman has been off duty. Should he sleep even a quarter of an hour during the night, it is pointed out on the Clock :—the Watchman is therefore compelled to be watchful. By this means the system of watching has been properly carried into effect. This Clock is one of the most ingenious contrivances you can imagine, and ensures watchfulness completely.

With your kind indulgence, I will trespass on your time and patience only a little longer, while I take a brief view of the *obstacles* to the practical execution of this, my theory. These obstacles do not arise from the nature of the cases—no, not in any one instance : neither are they in any instance *insurmountable.* What then are they ? *First.* The expense

of providing a Building having suitable apartments, Galleries, Dormitories, separate Sleeping Rooms, with Airing Courts, Pleasure
Grounds, Gardens, and Walks :—and such
ample remuneration of Attendants, as may
ensure persons of character and respectability.
But here it may be truly said, 'If a thing is
worth doing at all, it is worth doing well!'
If it be worth while to provide an Asylum
for the Insane, it is worth while also to render
that Asylum complete for its purposes; otherwise the main objects of the Charity, viz.—
the restoration of the afflicted inmates to sanity
or providing for their comfort if irrecoverable
—fall at once to the ground, and the Asylum
becomes a mere prison.

Secondly. The prejudice which this plan
(as has been the case with every improvement
on its first introduction) has to encounter.
*What! Let loose a Madman! Why he will
tear us to pieces!* Look a moment at the
facts. The following Table, conjoined with
the fact, that no serious accident has occurred
under this System, will I think, remove this
idea from the mind of any impartial person.
(See Table in the Appendix D.)

On comparing this Table with the Tables
of Restraints, and from a knowledge of the

circumstance that an effective system of Watch-fulness has only been introduced into the Asy-lum within the two or three last years,—it will appear that, without such a system of Watch-fulness,

A maximum of Restraints is more safe than a medium.

With such a system of Watchfulness, a minimum of Restraints is more safe than either.

It must be borne in mind, that the attend-ants are or should be tall, and powerful in appearance. A diminutive person would be liable to be attacked : not so with the former ; for a lunatic is perfectly aware (as is a sane person) with whom he has to deal. The attendants should be able to keep control with-out even the appearance of anger, and their demeanour and directions should be firm and decisive : nevertheless, this firmness must be always tempered with kindness ; for a maniac may be drawn, when ill usage would but irri-tate him. I have never at any time had the slightest difficulty in calming a patient when he has been apparently in a state bordering on violence. I have been threatened several times, but never met with any injury. I have always been able to withdraw their attention, and they have generally afterwards expressed their regret for any roughness of their conduct towards me. One or two kind expressions I have generally found sufficient to assuage any feelings of anger or of violence; and much will always depend on the demeanour of the Superintendent, as well as of the attendants.

Thirdly. The unwillingness of attendants, nurses, &c., to undertake the increased trouble, which this system requires. Here I have found my greatest difficulty; and I know of no way of surmounting it, except by an ample remuneration of such persons. It is stated truly in the Report of this year, that " it is in the power of an unwilling officer to make any improvements fail in practice." When a patient is under Restraint, it saves them the trouble of watching him : they can enjoy themselves at leisure, and play at cards, or otherwise amuse themselves as they please. Such was the case formerly, but cannot be tolerated under the new system. Their whole time and attention are now required for the patients.

I protest therefore, beforehand, against any failure in practice arising from unwillingness, inexperience, want of address, or impatience, on the part of any Officer, being converted

into an argument against the system. Failures,
if any should occur, will arise from one or
other of the above causes, and not from the
impracticability of the system itself. If others
should not succeed in pursuing this plan, I
shall have no fear of failure myself; as I feel
confident that with a properly constructed
building, and a sufficient number of tall, strong,
well-remunerated, and *willing* attendants, I
could introduce and act upon the system in
any Asylum in the kingdom.

Shall then a plan, which has for its object
the amelioration of the condition of an afflicted
class of our fellow-creatures, and a more humane treatment of them, together with a better
prospect of restoring them to the possession of
that noblest gift of God, without which man
sinks into a more abject state of misery and
degradation than the beasts which perish—
shall such a plan want advocates? I know
it will not. I feel confident that it only requires to be made known, to be duly appreciated. Shew its success, and humanity will
compel its adoption. The Legislature of our
Country deem not the welfare, the comfort,
and happiness of any portion of the people,
a subject unworthy of its consideration : and
if instruments of cruelty are in the habitations

which assume the names of a Refuge, an
Asylum, a Retreat from misery and woe, let
the Government, (when convinced of its practicability) banish them by law for ever! Let
not the deeds done in an Asylum, render its
very name a mockery. Let it be indeed a
Refuge from distress; an Asylum, not in name,
but in deed and in truth :—a place where the
sufferer may be shielded from injury and in-
sult—where his feelings may not be uselessly
wounded, nor his innocent wishes wantonly
thwarted. Here let him seek, and seek not
in vain, that peace and comfort which are
denied him in the paths he has formerly trod.
Here let him repose until the light begin to
dawn on his benighted mind, and he confess
with heartfelt joy and gratitude, that the day
he entered a Lunatic Asylum was indeed a
blessed day !

On the conclusion of the Lecture, the President of the Mechanics' Institution, Sir E.
Ff. Bromhead, Bart., F.R.S., L. and E., who
is also a Vice-President of the Lincoln Asylum,
offered some illustrative remarks on the sub-

ject of the Lecture, confirmatory of his own observation at the Asylum, of the soundness of the no-restraint theory. He then submitted to the meeting a formal vote of thanks to the Lecturer, which was carried in a manner most truly gratifying to his feelings.

APPENDIX.

A.

PROCEEDINGS

OF THE

LINCOLN LUNATIC ASYLUM,

RELATIVE TO CLASSIFICATION, INSPECTION, AND OTHER MATTERS BEARING
UPON THE SUBJECT OF RESTRAINT.

Extracts from the Original Rules.

1819. *Rule 44.*—That no forcible means be employed
in administering medicines to the patients, without specific
orders from the Physicians.

Rule 75.—That the attendants and servants never presume to use any degree of restraint or violence, without the
consent of the Director.

Extract from the House Visitor's Report.

1821, *March 5.*—In the course of the two last days, a
violent patient has broken three of the doors, one of which
is totally shattered. This is not the first occurrence of the
kind. The Director again requests me to express his conviction of the absolute and immediate necessity of fitting up
some of the cells, so as to render them capable of securing

powerful and violent patients. The circumstances which occurred yesterday will demonstrate to the Board the reasonableness and justness of this request.

Number of Patients—Males 6, Females 5.

(Signed) H. V. BAYLEY, Visitor.

1821, *March 5.*—Ordered, That Mr. Willson be desired to make the end cell in the Noisy Patients' Lower Gallery secure, for the safety of a powerful and violent Patient.

March 28.—Ordered, That two doors of the cells in the Upper Gallery for male patients, be secured in the same manner as those below, [i. e. with massive bolts and iron facings.]

August 20.—Order for an estimate of a wooden fence, to be five feet high, round the front grounds, on account of the escape of a patient.

Physician's Report.

1821, *October* 21.—No. —. I shall here observe that from the present very insecure state of the Asylum for want of an outer wall of sufficient height to prevent escapes, this and other patients are kept almost constantly fettered : it is not safe to allow them exercise even in the inner yards, except in that state : while the garden and front ground are rendered useless, not only to them but to the majority of the patients. Their comforts and the hopes of their recovery are thus so greatly abridged, that I cannot but request the earnest attention of the Governors to this point, as affecting the main interests of the Institution. I trust that they will see the necessity of appropriating the earliest accumulation of the funds to this object, by finishing the outer back (the garden) wall, and building a low wall round the front ground with a deep sunk fence within.

(Signed) E. P. CHARLESWORTH,

[Physician of the Month.]

House Visitor's Report.

1821, *October* 22.—I have visited the Asylum frequently in the course of the last week, and as far as the economy of the house is concerned, I see no cause of complaint myself, and hear of none either from the Director or the Matron; the provisions are very good, and every thing appears orderly and regular. But the attending Physician and the Director having both of them made the strongest representations to me of the insecurity of the building, from the inadequate state of the fences, I feel it my duty to submit the subject to the consideration of the Board: it is one which I am well aware has already often engaged their attention, and that pecuniary difficulties alone have prevented the adoption of some remedy for the evil complained of: but when I am expressly informed that owing to its continuance the patients are either prevented from taking the exercise proper for them, or in order to allow of their doing so without danger of escape, are fettered in a way which would be otherwise unnecessary, that their health from this cause is in many instances suffering, and their recovery in consequence retarded: and when it is evident that the character and credit of the Institution must be materially injured, if the idea of its insecurity is suffered to gain ground, I trust I shall stand excused for thus pressing the subject again on the notice of the Board.

Number of Patients—Males 11, Females 3.

(Signed)   GEORGE GORDON, [Visitor.]

October 29.—Ordered, That an estimate be given of a wall round the front ground, with a sunk fence within.

Extract from the Physician's Report.

1821, *December* 4.—No. — is seldom quiet for more than an hour together throughout the day, and is a perpetual source of disturbance to the other patients.

This case and many others call upon me to express my regret, at the very limited means which the Institution affords for Classing the patients. At present the Epileptic, the Melancholic, the Idiotic, the Incurable, and the Convalescent all associate together, with no other separation than what is determined by their respective payments. That such an arrangement is not calculated to restore disordered minds, must strike the most common observer : and that it is contrary to the practice and experience of other Institutions, is fully shewn in the numerous enlightened Reports which are now before the public.

I am aware that the necessary improvements cannot be effected in the present exhausted state of the finances. On them however, the character and support of the Institution must eventually rest, as involving the security, the health, and the restoration of the patients, who for want of them are on many occasions confined with chains, take exercise in damp dull yards, and associate in a manner calculated to obstruct their cure.

(Signed)　　　　E. P. CHARLESWORTH,

[Physician of the Month.]

1822, *April* 10.—Ordered, That the garden walls be raised four feet.

[About this period various estimates were from time to time ordered.]

October 28.—Resolved, That it is the opinion of this Board that a general boundary wall is now become a matter of imperious necessity.

That William Fotherby's proposal for building such boundary wall, to be ten feet high round the ground in front of the Asylum, be accepted : that the work be proceeded with as soon as the season of the year will permit.

Extract from the Physician's Report.

1823, *February* 28.—I once more wish to press upon the attention of the Governors the expediency of taking measures for Classing the patients.

The Association of the men has now become so insupportably inconvenient, that some of them are kept almost constantly in manacles, or apart in the maniacal cells, to protect the weak and quiet from the outrages of the strong: (see occasional Reports of the Physician and of the Director.)

(*Signed*) E. P. CHARLESWORTH,
[Physician of the Month.]

House Visitor's Report.

1823, *March* 3.—I beg to observe that two patients of the names of —— and —— were confined in irons, the former by having an iron bar between his legs, (of which he complained very much,) which prevented his closing them together; and the other by having his hands confined by handcuffs, and were with the other patients in the Gallery. I therefore thought proper to enquire the reason of their being so confined, when I was informed that —— was always tearing his clothes and pulling the other patients about, and that —— was in the habit of breaking the windows. I therefore think it right to mention this circumstance as a corroborating proof how necessary it is in my opinion, (with deference to that of others,) and how desirable it would be, if a Classification could be made.

Number of Patients—Men 17, Women 4.

(*Signed*) JOHN FARDELL, [Visitor.]

House Visitor's Report.

1823, *October* 13.—With the means of accommodation, which the Asylum at present affords, every thing seems going on as successfully as can in reason be expected. The enclosure of the Front Area now nearly completed, will bring into use a piece of ground of incalculable value to the uses of the Institution. And nothing further will then appear to be wanting but increased facilities for Classification, which, as being of the utmost importance to the best interests of the charity, it is much to be wished its funds may soon be in a state to furnish the means of supplying.

Number of Patients—Males 17, Females 4.

(Signed)   George Gordon, [Visitor.]

[After this, various plans with a view to Classification were proposed, and discussed by the Board.]

1827, *April* 28.—Resolved, That a Committee consisting of the Dean, the Mayor, Sir E. Ff. Bromhead, Bart., the Precentor, Major King, Dr. Cookson,* Dr. Charlesworth, and Mr. Alderman Snow, be a Committee to carry into effect the Plan now produced and signed by the Chairman, or any part of it; or to vary it at their discretion, taking care to connect the noisy cells with the main building in the first instance.

Resolved, That the thanks of this meeting be given to Dr. Charlesworth for the plan produced by him this day and approved.

October 3.—A report from the Building Committee being read,

Resolved, That the said report is hereby approved and confirmed, and that the same be entered on the minutes.

Extracts from the Report.

The committee appointed to carry into effect the Plan approved of by the last special general meeting, have pro-

---

* Dr. Cookson resigned his seat on the Committee, at the following Board.

ceeded, as far as the means placed at their disposal would allow. They have formed the department for the insensible and noisy male patients, and have connected it with the main building, as was especially prescribed.

On the female side, both the proposed new building and the alterations of the house may be postponed, as the small number of patients does not in so pressing a manner call for a change.—

Extracts from the General Remarks.

The means of Classing the patients generally or according to circumstances will be effectually provided.

The Upper Rank patients will be brought from the back to the front of the building, and

The Insensible and Noisy patients will be removed from the front to the back.

The Convalescents will be separated from both, and will not be placed in Galleries but in Rooms, which do not present any appearance of confinement.

The distinctions [of Rank] will be more rigidly observed as the patients approach to Convalescence and as they become more sensible of such distinctions.

The Kitchen and Noisy Cells being removed from the front to the rear, will render the whole south front of the building available for the enjoyment of the patients.

Those Offices which give employment to the Female patients, will be attached to the Female side of the building.

The Airing Courts will be greatly enlarged and will extend beyond the shade of the building.

The front ground will be rendered sufficiently private, and the patients will not see their friends approaching the house, which is often improper.

1828, *October* 13.—At a General Board of Governors, Edward Wright, Esq., *in the Chair*, Sir Edward Ffrench Bromhead, Bart., V.P., the Very Rev. the Dean of Lincoln, V.P., the Worshipful the Mayor of Lincoln, Charles Mainwaring, Esq., *Treasurer*, E. P. Charlesworth, M.D., Charles Beaty, M.D., Henry Hutton, Esq., *Auditor*, John Fardell, Esq., *Auditor*, William Burton Burton, Esq., Mr. Alderman Snow, *Surgeon.*

A Letter from one of the Physicians of the Asylum was read:

Extracts from the Letter.

" My jealousy on the point of facility of inspection is extreme. Viewing this privilege, qualified as it is by our rules, as one of the principal safeguards of the patients, I regard every step towards its diminution as a step towards maltreatment, and every impediment thrown in its way as introductory to abuse. In these sentiments, and in the opinion derived from practical observation, that insane patients are very rarely indeed excited by inspection, I will endeavour to show that I am supported by the published experience of different asylums, and by other respectable authorities. * * *

"Whenever the domestic officers of an establishment are ill-disposed, or overbearing, or indolent, or for any other reason averse from observation, specious arguments will be found to preserve their domain from intruding eyes as much as possible. And so long as the formal words ' improper to be seen ' are to be accepted as an unquestionable reason for shrouding from inspection, even of the weekly-appointed* visitors, any insane patient to whom they are applied, a con-

* " It is superfluous to mention the extreme danger of any mistaken delicacy in the Official Guardians of the Patients, with regard to a personal inspection of their condition."

venient cloak will be ever at hand to cover any severity, neglect, or other abuse.

" The seeds of abuse exist in every institution : and the example of other asylums has painfully shown how difficult they are to be eradicated when they have once taken root; and how governors the most honorable and humane may be drawn into a misplaced confidence. Even respectable persons may, by habit, become reconciled to spectacles, which would startle a stranger, and which could not, for a moment, be endured under the public eye.

" From the peculiar nature of an asylum for the insane, the most horrible abuses may exist within its walls without suspicion, and almost without the possibility of detection. Sir Andrew Halliday has observed, ' *The mystery which has been made to hover round the precincts of a mad-house, was sufficient to baffle common enquiry; and the utter seclusion so insidiously inculcated, made it next to impossible to discover the scenes of horror that took place within its walls.*' Hence our attention should ever be directed to a system of *prevention*, which can be rendered effectual only by keeping our grounds, courts, galleries, cells, offices, and as much as possible, the persons of the patients, open to that rational inspection, which our rules have provided for, and which general experience has shown to be safe as well as necessary.

" The surest evidence of the good conduct of any establishment, is its facility of access.* No consideration should induce the managers of a *public* asylum to receive any patients, whose friends show a disposition to obstruct governors and persons officially introduced, in the full and free inspection necessary for the prevention of abuses; such as foul,

---

* " Well-disposed Officers will be found invariably to court inspection : they feel a pride in the cleanliness, good order, and kind treatment, which are instantly visible to an intelligent observer."

offensive, and unventilated apartments, personal uncleanness
and neglect, brutal means of restraint, harsh unfeeling demeanour in the attendants, and above all, improper association in convalescence. Persons highly sensitive on the point
of inspection should send their unhappy relatives to some
distant institution, where their persons are not known, or
should place them under private care. High payments cannot compensate a public asylum for the admission of cases
offering so dangerous an apology for closed doors. If we
permit one step to be taken in the road to concealment,
another will soon follow, till in the end the eyes even of the
governors themselves shall be deemed an intrusion, and their
enquiries be treated as an offensive evidence of distrust.

" These observations, which apply rather to public institutions, such as the Lincoln Asylum, than to private establishments, are of course not intended to recommend any meddling
interference with the patients. The inspection should extend
only to prevent personal ill-treatment ; and no stranger
should be permitted to address them, or to make any audible
remarks in their presence ; strangers visiting the institution
should be cautioned upon these points.

" E. P. CHARLESWORTH, M.D."

Ordered and Resolved, [on the motion of Sir E. Ff.
Bromhead, Bart., seconded by the Very Rev. the Dean,]

That the said letter be entered on the minutes of this
Board.

That this Board highly approves the sound principles
contained in the said letter, and will see the same carried
into full effect in this Asylum; and that the Director, Matron,
and other officers, be strictly enjoined to give their best
attention therein.

That the Lincoln Lunatic Asylum is a Public Institution,
and not a private establishment; and that no patients be

admitted on any terms however liberal, where the friends show a disposition to impede the inspection necessary for the prevention of abuses.

That the flagrant abuses lately brought to light before Parliament, such as foul, offensive, and unventilated apartments ; personal uncleanliness and neglect ; brutal means of restraint ; harsh unfeeling demeanour in the attendants ; and above all, improper association in convalescence ; never can be effectually prevented without a full and free inspection by governors, and strangers officially introduced.

That at each Quarterly Board, before the commencement of the ordinary business, the governors present be requested to inspect the building, and see every patient.

That a copy of Rule XXIV. as below stated,* and of Rule XXIII.† be conspicuously placed in the principal entrance ; and that a note be subjoined thereto, requesting strangers not to address the patients, or make any audible remarks in their presence ; and that strangers be further requested to write in the Book, before the entry of their names, any improvements which they can suggest, or any abuses which they may observe, or any incivility or want of attention to themselves, and especially any impediment to the full and free inspection of the Asylum.

That the " Strangers' Memorandum Book" do lie on the table in the principal entrance, and that a Plan of the Asylum

---

* Rule 24.—" That it is desirable that every proper facility be given to inspect this Establishment, so that its real state may be at all times ascertained, and its regulations carried into effect ; but at the same time care must be taken, that it be not exposed, for the gratification of idle curiosity, to the interruption of order, and the prejudice of the Patients."

† Rule 23.—" That no person residing in the Asylum do at any time presume to give to or take from any Tradesman, Patient or Servant, Stranger, or other person whatsoever, any Fee, Reward, or Gratuity, directly or indirectly, for any service done or to be done on account of the Asylum, on pain of expulsion."

be there hung up, to enable them to ascertain whether any part of the building has been concealed from inspection.

That every instrument of restraint, without exception, *when not in use*, be hung up in a place distinctly appropriated in some easily accessible part of the Asylum, so that the *number in use at any time*, the nature of such instruments, and their state of cleanliness, may appear; and that the Director and Matron be enjoined to enforce a strict observance of this regulation from the keepers and nurses.

That the Physicians be requested to consider, whether it be possible to make any improvement in the means of restraint now in use, and especially for obviating the use of the strait-waistcoat.

That any Governor may inspect, extract, or copy, any bills, accounts, vouchers, registers, documents, and minute books, provided that the names of the patients shall not be copied.

(Signed)   EDWARD WRIGHT, Chairman.

House Visitor's Report.

1828, *December* 1.—On visiting the Asylum this week, I have witnessed with the highest satisfaction the important advantages resulting from the recent improvements: from what has been already done, the benefits expected are largely experienced, and will be still more fully felt when the remaining alterations are completed; I observed the same attention as usual to cleanliness and order, and the provisions of every sort appeared to be good.

Number of Patients—Males 25, Females 20.

(Signed)   GEO. GORDON, [Visitor.]

1829, *February* 16.—Resolved, That it appears to this Board, after full enquiry, that —— died in consequence of being strapped to the bed in a strait-waistcoat during the night.

Ordered, That the use of the Strait-Waistcoat be discontinued in this Institution, except under the special written order of the Physician of the Month; and that an Attendant do continue in the room all night, whenever its use during the night shall be ordered.

That the Director do keep a Journal, in which he shall make daily entry of every Restraint and Severity used in this Institution, specifying the Name of the patient, the Nature of the restraint or severity applied, and the Hours at which the same commenced and ended; and that the said Journal be laid before each Weekly Board, and signed by the Chairman.

1829, *April* 8.—Ordered, That where any peculiar circumstance makes it improper that a patient should be seen, the Director shall enter the circumstance with his reason in his Journal, whether any Stranger enter a complaint or not; and that the House Visitor and Physician do at their next visit see such patient, and enter the Patients' State in their Books and Journal.

*Extracts from the Fifth Report of the
Lincoln Lunatic Asylum.*

1829, *April.*—During the last session of Parliament two important Acts were passed, consolidating the whole of the existing law concerning Lunatic Asylums, and introducing a great variety of improvements for the prevention of abuses.

When the bills were first brought into Parliament, they contained a variety of clauses for the visitation and control of Public Asylums. These clauses were dropped in the progress of the bills through Parliament; and it has been the feeling of the Governors of this Institution, that this confidence so liberally placed in them by the Legislature, should be met by every possible exertion on their part to adopt the views of Parliament as far as applicable. It may indeed be

laid down as a principle in human nature, which experience
will amply confirm, that no Institution of this sort can be
considered safe in its management, where the Managers are
not subject to some eye unconnected with the government of
the Institution itself. The Public eye and Public opinion
have in all cases been found the most efficient; and the
original Rules of this Institution, wisely and humanely acting
upon this principle, court and avow a system of Public
Inspection under due regulation. This same principle the
Governors have now further pursued, by endeavouring to
give additional facility to the observation of the state of the
Patients and of the Institution, by all the respectable classes
of society. At the same time they have opened a second
entrance to the Asylum, by which they have prevented all
persons approaching the house merely on business, from
passing continually through the very midst of the Patients,
in their principal exercise ground as heretofore : and have
also taken means to prevent Strangers from addressing the
Patients, or even making remarks in their presence, by
placing them under the care of a responsible officer, while
passing through the wards. Every opportunity is afforded
to all who inspect the Asylum, to record any observations
and suggestions they may think proper to make; and where,
in any case, peculiarity in the disease may imperatively require privacy, the Director is fully authorized to prevent
inspection in such case ; under this condition however, that
he is required to lay all the circumstances of the case before
the proper authorities without delay, in order to secure from
abuse this hazardous though necessary discretion.*

* " A Lunatic Asylum is unlike every other establishment for the care or
" confinement of human beings, in this respect, that the Patients are wholly in-
" competent witnesses, and too often that there is no direct mode of detecting
" any fault in their treatment, but through those who have an interest in con-
" cealing it."

13th Report of the Glasgow Asylum, p. 9.

The Governors have particularly directed their views to the subject of Coercion and Restraints, well aware of their injurious consequences to the Patients, and seeing from the late Parliamentary investigations on these points, the deplorable results which caprice, tyranny, negligence, and above all a wish to avoid necessary attention and trouble, have elsewhere produced. In order to ascertain the number and condition of the Instruments in use for these purposes, instead of being dispersed in all parts of the house under the control of the inferior Keepers as heretofore, they are now collected in a single apartment, accessible at once, and open to inspection at any moment. In the next place, the Governors have adopted a Register universally used in the Scotch Asylums, wherein the Director is bound to enter the Nature of every instance of restraint, and the Time of its continuance, during the night as well as the day. And lastly, the construction of the instruments in use having also been carefully examined, they have destroyed a considerable proportion of those, that were not of the most improved and least irritating description, and hope hereafter to introduce still further amelioration into this department.——

(*Signed*)　　R. Prettyman,
　　　　　　　　Chairman.

1829, *May* 4.—Ordered, That the heaviest pair of iron Hobbles* and the heaviest pair of iron Handcuffs,† be destroyed.

That of the eleven Strait-waistcoats now belonging to the House, the worst five be destroyed.

The Director having stated to this Board, that in the case of ——, it is essentially necessary that he should have a Belt in the Nurse's Room:—Ordered that he be authorised to remove one there accordingly.

* Jointed: weight 3lbs. 8oz.　　　† Solid: weight 1lb. 5oz.

Extract from the House Visitor's Report.

1829, *June* 1.—It is pleasing to find that the more violent
and noisy [Male] Patients are now inhabiting their own
Gallery, with its cheerful airing ground adjoining; and I
could not but observe a forcible illustration of the great advantage of a proper Classification, in the comparative quiet
and comfort which pervade the Male department. One excellent room in front, ready for the reception of any of them,
is as yet unoccupied, which I presume will not long remain
so : but with respect to the Female side, a common observer
like myself must naturally wish that the keeping together
such a mixture of the opposite characters of Insanity, as is
now to be seen in one Gallery, could by any possibility be
avoided.—After a consideration of the fact that first Class
Patients bear no proportion in numbers to the rest, I have
no hesitation in expressing my decided conviction that they
are not kept away by the rule to which this absence has been
attributed : and, while expressing my sentiments upon this
subject, I will go so far as to state, that even if I believed,
which I do not, that the system of Inspection was generally
objected to by the public, I could not bring myself to consent
to its abolition; being firmly persuaded that in all Lunatic
Asylums, the eye of the Public is the only real and solid security against harsh treatment, unnecessary restraint, or
improper absence of responsible attendants. The same dis-
proportion of wealthy Patients is to be seen at York, where
their department is strictly private; and it is clear to me
from observation, as well as from the constitution of human
nature, that whatever separation may be made, or whatever
advantages may be held out, there is a prejudice in the higher
ranks of life against all Lunatic Asylums, which are indis-
criminately open to the rich and poor.

(Signed)   R. PRETYMAN, [Visitor.]

Extracts from the House Visitor's Report.

1829, *August* 17.—Every attention seems to be paid to the Patients, whose general state has I understand, for some time past, been so generally good, that it is gratifying to say the Strait-Waistcoat has almost become useless.

Number of Patients—Males 29, Females 13.

(*Signed*) HENRY HUTTON, [Visitor.]

1829, *September* 21.—The Director having applied for a Belt and a pair of Hobbles to be placed in the Keeper's room in the North Gallery, on account of some of the Patients, who are subject to sudden fits of violence :—Ordered that a Belt and Hobbles be placed there accordingly.

October 19.—Ordered, That whenever the Director thinks it essentially necessary to place any Instruments of Restraint at the disposal of the inferior Keepers, he shall enter the Number and Place on Saturday at the foot of his Journal of Restraints, taking the opinion of the Board or Physician when practicable.

1829, *November* 30. — Ordered, That the Director's " Journal," " Register of Restraints," and " Register of Persons daily maintained" be made up by him not later than ten o'clock in the morning for the day and night preceding.

1830, *November* 29.—Ordered, That the Director have power to procure List-shoes for any patient, who he has reason to think would do injury with his feet.

Extract from the Seventh Annual Report.

1831, *March* 28.—A new Director* has also been elected, in recording whose appointment, the Governors would not do justice either to their own feelings or to his merits, if they did not bear a willing testimony to the zeal and fidelity,

* Mr. Henry Marston.

with which he discharges the various duties of his office. A circumstance this, abundantly proving what it is of public importance to know, that there is not anything in the Office of Director of a Lunatic Asylum, for which any gentleman of professional talent, firmness, and good temper, may not be deemed fully qualified. The greatest advantage may be expected from this Office being thrown open to the general competition of the Profession, instead of being confined to a limited and exclusive part of it.

Heretofore it was conceived that the only intention of a receptacle for the Insane, was the safe custody of the unhappy objects, by any means however harsh and severe. These views are now passing away, and the fair measure of a Superintendent's ability in the treatment of such patients, will be found in the small number of Restraints which are imposed. The new Director has answered this test in a very satisfactory manner.*

(Signed)   GEORGE GORDON,

Chairman.

July 13.—Ordered, That the Weekly Visitor be requested to examine the Instruments of Restraint, and remove such as are improper.

October 24.—Ordered, That the Instruments of Restraint now produced, be destroyed. That the leathern straps and the buckles on the strait-waistcoats, be replaced by ties.

That a very strong leathern body-belt be procured.

That the Instruments of Restraint be put into a state of thorough repair weekly, and well cleaned every Saturday, and shewn to the Weekly Visitor.

---

* As early as the 24th day of November last, there was not any patient in the house, out of forty-eight, under restraint, unless one wearing a collar, which leaves all the limbs quite at liberty, can be so considered. This gratifying occurrence has taken place more than once since that time.

Extract from the Eighth Annual Report.

1832, *March* 26.—The Register of Restraints shows a continued diminution in their number. Strangers who derive their notions of an Asylum from the coloured pictures of imaginative writers, or from ill-conducted establishments where severity is made to supersede vigilance and attention, are surprised at the freedom, repose, and cheerfulness, which appear through the whole house. The Boards have kept steadily in view the Nature of the Restraints employed, and have great pleasure in having been able to destroy several Instruments of a coarse and harsh construction, which an exaggerated caution had originally provided, and which experience has proved to be unnecessary.——

(Signed)   E. P. CHARLESWORTH,

Chairman.

[*Extracts from the Revised Rules.*]

1832, *April* 11.

OCCASIONAL VISITING.

Persons wishing to visit the Asylum, may be personally introduced by one of the Physicians, Surgeons, or Governors, or by the written order of a Governor; and the House-Surgeon may admit any respectable non-resident of Lincoln to see the establishment, without a special order.

The Ordinary Board may exclude any individual Visitant by a special order on their minutes.

Visitants shall in all cases be accompanied by a Physician, or the House-Surgeon, or Matron, and shall be cautioned not to address the Patients, nor make any audible remark in their presence, without express permission; and on every such occasion, where any peculiar circumstance makes it necessary that a Patient shall be secluded, the House-Surgeon shall enter the circumstance, as a remarkable occurrence, with his reasons in his Journal.

A " Strangers' Memorandum Book" shall lie on the table in the Principal Entrance, and the names and address of all Visitants, with the name of the person introducing them, shall be entered. A Plan of the Building shall be there hung up, so that no part thereof can be concealed; and Visitants shall be requested to write in the Book before the entry of their names, any improvement which they can suggest, or any abuses which they may observe, or any incivility or want of attention to themselves, and especially any impediment to the full and free inspection of the Asylum.

COERCION, RESTRAINT.

One or two places shall be appropriated, in some easily accessible part of the Asylum, for the Instruments of Restraint, which shall be there hung up and numbered, so that the nature of such instruments, their state of repair and cleanliness, and also the number actually applied, or in the keeping of the Attendants for any emergency, may appear; and no new instrument shall be procured without the order of the Board.

The House-Surgeon shall reduce the number kept by the attendants for emergencies, as low as possible, and shall state the number so appropriated every Saturday at the foot of his " Register of Restraints," for the information and sanction of the Physician and the Boards.

No Attendant, on pain of dismissal, shall strike any Patient, except in urgent self-defence; nor apply any force, restraint, or privation, without the House-Surgeon's order, except on emergency. The Attendant shall give instant information to the House-Surgeon for power to continue any Restraint or Privation, which shall, in all cases, be as moderate as is consistent with safety.

No forcible means shall be employed in giving food or

medicine to any Patient, without a special order in the Physician's Journal in each case.

The Strait-Waistcoat shall not be used in this Institution, without the special written order of the Physician in his Journal, on each occasion; and an Attendant shall continue in the room all night, whenever its use in the night shall be so ordered.

The House-Surgeon shall keep a " Register of Restraints," in which he shall make daily entry of every Coercion, Restraint, and Severity, practised in this Institution, and shall specify the Nature thereof, the Name of the Patient, and the Hours at which the same commenced and ended; and the said Register shall be laid weekly before the Board, and signed by the Chairman in proof thereof.

MORAL TREATMENT.

The Patients shall be treated with all the forbearance, mildness, and indulgence, compatible with steady and effectual control.

No Attendant or other person shall attempt to deceive or terrify any Patient, or violate any promise made; nor presume to irritate any Patient by incivility, disrespect, contempt, mockery, mimicry, or sarcasm; nor use wanton allusions to any thing ridiculous or degrading in the present appearance or past conduct of the Patient; nor swear, nor address any Patient with a raised voice or in an imperious tone; nor conduct themselves towards any of the Patients in such a manner as to excite envy, jealousy, or ill-will among the rest; nor shall they dispute or argue with them, or needlessly contradict them; nor shall they indulge or express vindictive feelings, but considering the Patients as if unable to restrain themselves, shall forgive all petulance or abuse, and treat with equal kindness those who give the most trouble, and those who give the least.

The Attendants shall not unnecessarily converse with the non-convalescent patients, and shall speak principally in reply only, and shall especially avoid the subject of the Patient's delusion. They shall not incautiously speak of any Patients in their presence, nor on the subject of Insanity, nor unnecessarily do any act, the remembrance of which may be hurtful to any Patient's feelings on Convalescence.

Such Occupation and Amusement as may employ the time, divert the mind, win the attention, and awaken the affections, shall be cheerfully and readily promoted; and the Boards shall direct books of Prints, Chess, &c., with Periodicals and other light reading, to be supplied for Patients competent thereto.

1832, *July* 16.—Ordered, That Buckskin, and round cornered Buckles be used for the Hobbles.

That a leathern Belt for temporary security of patients becoming suddenly violent, be kept in the attendants' rooms.

That two strong Dresses be procured for the Male patients, who tear their clothes.

July 23.—Resolved, That a pair of quarter Boots* [of ticking] with rings fixed to the soles, be procured as a night restraint for patients requiring the same [instead of the Hobbles.]

Extract from the House Visitor's Report.

December 10.—I cannot help observing that a House-Porter appears to be much wanted in this Institution, to undertake the mowing, gardening, carrying messages, cleaning windows, and various other domestic occupations, which

----

* This mild substitute for the use of the ordinary Hobbles during the night, was suggested by Dr. Charlesworth.

at present appear to interfere too much with the business of the keepers.

Number of Patients—Males 37, Females 13.

(Signed)   Geo. Marr, [Visitor.]

Extract from the Physician's Report.

1832, *July* 31.—I have had occasion to remark in this month upon the case of a patient kept under continual Restraint on account of the insecurity of the inner Male court. This inconvenience has been met, it is hoped effectually, by a slight alteration of the windows of the adjoining Gallery, which had afforded a passage to the roof.

An order has been made by the Board to procure "strong Dresses" for patients disposed to tear their clothes. The intention is, by the use of these and the ordinary "Belt," to obviate the necessity of the "Muff," an instrument of restraint against which several serious objections exist. A principal defect is that it prevents the wearer from attending to the common calls of nature, occasioning not only much present suffering, but often entailing incurable disease and the most loathsome habits.

The Board has also ordered a substitute for the "Hobbles" employed to confine the feet of very violent patients during the night. The straps and buckles forming this instrument, were found to cause severe and injurious pressure under the unrelaxing strain which such patients will frequently exert, regardless or insensible of the injurious consequences.

It should be a fixed principle in the construction of *all* instruments of restraint, to prevent as much as possible the capability of the patients to effect any injurious change of their position, or otherwise to increase their severity. An insane patient will act, while under a paroxysm, not only as if he were insensible of pain, but even as if he preferred a state of suffering which would be found intolerable under ordinary circumstances. Multiplied instances, some of them very extraordinary, could be produced in proof; and the pathological inductions to which this fact would appear to lead, may perhaps hereafter throw additional light upon the medical history of Insanity.

With regard to the "fixing on" of the instruments of restraint, nothing can prevent the dangers of negligence on the part of the Attendants in securing the locks, or *what is much more common, the distressing severity of over caution in tightening the straps, &c.*, except minute and continually repeated personal examination by the superiour officers in each individual instance, and especially of the cases left for the night.

(Signed)   E. P. CHARLESWORTH,
                [Attending Physician.]

1833, *March* 11.—Ordered, That an additional servant be engaged as assistant in the Laundry, instead of hiring occasional assistance as heretofore, and allowing the Female servants and attendants to wash their own clothes.

Extracts from the Ninth Annual Report.

1833, *April.*—The Boards have pleasure in being able to state that the recent alterations in the Buildings and Courts are found to answer all the intentions of the Governors. The experience both of the past and present arrangements has fully confirmed the following observation of MR. TUKE, in his "*Remarks on the Construction of Public Institutions for the Cure of Mental Derangement:*" "However desirable a good system of management may be, no such system can be prosecuted with effect in an ill-contrived building. The defects of arrangement must unavoidably affect the Patient, and operate both against his comfort and cure." He adds, that they are " productive of evils, to which no management can oppose any adequate remedy."——

It is unceasingly an object in this Institution, and should form a prominent point in the Annual Reports, to dispense with or improve as much as possible the Instruments of Restraint. Nothing is more easy than to multiply ingenious inventions fully effectual for the direct purpose of confinement, but injurious as encouraging the system itself ; it has here, on the contrary, been the design to diminish the number of these instruments, and to simplify the construction, where vigilance and attention cannot wholly supply their place. Many restraints and privations, to the appearance of which custom has reconciled the Governors of receptacles for the Insane, as mere matters of course or of unavoidable necessity, might generally be traced to the principle of saving trouble to the attendants ; while the plausible ingenuity frequently displayed in obtaining that end, has been suffered to disguise its cruelty and injurious effects, and has contributed in no small degree to the popular delusion which prevails respecting the difficulty and " mystery" of managing the insane.

The propensity of some Patients to destroy their wearing apparel has been found a great inconvenience in all Asylums, and has introduced the use of the " Muff," an instrument open to some of the worst objections against the Strait-Waistcoat ;* but now nearly superseded in the Lincoln Asylum by adopting for such persons a dress which is not torn without great difficulty.—Some Patients so obstinately refuse food, that compulsory means are unavoidable, for which purpose practitioners have generally forced open the mouth and used a speculum or stomach pump, a method troublesome and sometimes dangerous. The Asylum is indebted to Mr. Bakewell of Spring Vale, among other

* See First Report of the Parliamentary Committee on Mad-houses, 1815, Mr. John Haslam's evidence, p. 63.

ingenious suggestions, for an instrument which has effectually superseded the above practice, by means of a tin vessel so contrived that the Patient, in the mere act of breathing, without having the teeth forced open, cannot resist the introduction of fluid nutriment.——

The Governors will have received copies of the Revised Rules, which were unanimously passed at a very numerous General Board after a minute examination. They have been founded on an extensive collation of the Rules of various Asylums, the works of writers on the subject, and the experience of this Institution itself. It is hoped that it may not be invidious to mention the liberal code of the Establishment at Aberdeen, as having afforded many useful suggestions.

(Signed)   John Wm. Sturges,
Chairman.

May 6.—Ordered, That the Fire-guards have the inner wiring continued throughout their whole surface.

May 13.—The House-Surgeon stated [to the Board] that the Keepers have not time to attend to the premises both within doors and without doors, without neglecting the patients.

May 20.—Ordered, That a man be engaged as House-Porter and Gardener, as a trial.

July 15.—That a Bell be fixed in the passage over the sitting room door of the House-Surgeon, and another over the door of the Matron, communicating with the Galleries on the Male and Female sides of the House respectively, to be rung by the Attendants on every occasion of necessity for restraint or other extraordinary circumstance happening among the Patients.

Physician's Report.

1834, *January* 31.—I will beg to call the attention of
the Board to the propriety of considering whether the use of
fermented liquors under the general diet table, should not be
discontinued, and the matter left for medical order in special
cases. It is very questionable whether the temporary tone
procured by any kind of stimulus, is not in many cases mischievous, and whether the curative process should not be
made to depend upon a permanent increase of tone indirectly
procured by nutrition, air, and exercise.

(Signed)   E. P. Charlesworth,
[Attending Physician.]

February 3.—Resolved, That the Physician's Report
relating to the Beer, be referred to the Physicians of this
Institution.

February 10.—In pursuance of a resolution at the last
weekly Board, that the opinion of the Physicians of this
Institution, [Dr. Charlesworth, Dr. W. Cookson, and Dr.
Elmhirst,] should be taken on the subject of discontinuing
the use of fermented liquors for the patients, except under
special medical order, and the Physicians having unanimously
recommended its dis-continuance.

Ordered, That the use of fermented liquor for the patients
of this Institution be dis-continued for the future, except under special medical order.

Extracts from the Tenth Annual Report.

1834, *March.*—Strangers who visit the Lincoln Lunatic
Asylum usually express their great surprise at the freedom
enjoyed by the patients, and the rarity of even individual
instances of personal restraint. The treatment by which
the patients are induced to supply by self-control the necessity
for restraint, may be explained partly by the facility, which

the improved construction of the building gives for the separation of the patients into appropriate Classes—partly by the liberty which the enlarged Airing Grounds allow for exercise and recreation—and especially by the absence of all those engagements on the part of the House-Surgeon and Attendants, which would divert them from the observation of the patients, or from a plea for the neglect of this their principal and special charge.——

It has long been considered an object in this Institution, not to attempt, either on the ground of economy or of profitable speculation, the production of any of the articles consumed. All such speculations, even if successful, must have the effect of occupying the time and attention of the Officers and Servants, and of adding a complexity to the management inconsistent with that close and unremitting observation, which an assemblage of insane persons, irresponsible for their conduct towards themselves or others, must constantly require: nor could even the employment, which might possibly be afforded to a portion of the patients from this source, be a counter-balance for the danger of neglecting the remainder. The experience of this Asylum has shown, that not more than a very few of the patients can be depended upon for the regular performance of even the simplest operations, such as digging, raking the borders of the shrubberies, rolling the walks, weeding, gathering stones, pumping water, helping in the house, needlework, &c., except under a superintendence which would preclude all pretensions to economy or profit, if hired for the purpose, or otherwise would leave patients unguarded, or safe only by personal restraint. The management of Cattle, the operations of Husbandry, and even Gardening if in any degree to be rendered a source of profit, have all fixed seasons for their performance, and cannot wait upon the will of persons subject to capricious variations of temper and capability; they must be executed under all the vicissitudes of the weather, and frequently require considerable judgment and practical knowledge merely to avoid loss.—There is not any intention in these remarks to undervalue the salutary effects of occupation or exercise, especially in the open air, avoiding severe labour, violent exertion, and perhaps also such employments as require a long continued stooping posture. These can however be obtained for the patients competent to them, in all Asylums where the Airing-grounds are of a reasonable size, by the ordinary cultivation which the pleasure-grounds demand, by the encouragement of various safe games and recreations, by the introduction of living animals whose habits are inoffensive and amusing, and by assisting in the household duties—without resorting to means, which may hazard the safety or abridge the liberty of the patients, or may risk in costly speculations the contributions of the charitable and the payments of the poor.

By a recent regulation the use of fermented liquor, as part of the regular diet, has been discontinued, except under medical order; while the diet table has in other respects been enlarged. It may be questionable whether the temporary tone procured by this stimulus, may not in many cases be mischievous. It is a safer practice to attempt the curative process, through a permanent increase of a healthy tone, indirectly procured by nutrition, air, and exercise; and it is especially important to establish, both as a principle and a habit, abstinence in a point, where excess has been found to be so eminently injurious to the insane, as well as to those predisposed to become so, and to be such a frequent cause of relapse.

(*Signed*)   Thos. Brailsford, **Chairman.**

Physician's Report.

1834, *July* 1.—As the disposition of some of the Patients to tear their blankets is occasionally a cause of their being confined by the wrists at night, I would recommend that in such cases, the blankets should be inclosed within strong Russia sheeting, quilted.

(*Signed*) E. P. Charlesworth,

[Attending Physician.]

1834, *July* 9.—Resolved, That the Weekly Board do take into consideration the propriety of a Night Watch.

That the Weekly Board do take measures for improving the system of Restraints, so as to prevent the injurious effects of confining the fingers of the patients.

July 21.—Ordered, That the Instruments* of Restraint now produced, being unnecessary, be destroyed.

Extract from the House Visitor's Report.

August 4 to 10 inclusive.—I have much satisfaction in being able to state that not a single Male patient has been under restraint since the 16th of July, and not one Female patient since the 1st of August, and then only for a few hours.

Number of Patients—Males 41, Females 18.

(*Signed,*) Henry Hutton, [Visitor.]

Extract from the House Visitor's Report.

August 11.—I have much pleasure in adding my testimony to that of the preceding Visitor, in approbation of the continued infrequency (as appears from the Register) of Instances of Restraint, Privation, or Severity. The House-Surgeon will of course see that his humane intentions in checking the use of Instruments, are not evaded by the substitution of a system of violence and intimidation on the part of the attendants, for their own ease.

* Strait-waistcoats, jacket and sleeves, muffs;—instruments which confine the fingers.

Examining the condition of the Instruments, and fitting of the attendants' keys, I have found them all quite clean, but several out of order as regards the locks and screws and keys. My notice of them would have led to their immediate regulation and repair, which is required to be attended to every Saturday : but I would beg first to suggest that such of the wristlocks as are fastened by the tedious process of screwing, should be laid aside and replaced by others acting with spring locks, constructed, if practicable, with the inner space made circular instead of oblong. This form would prevent the patients from inflicting intentional injury on themselves, as they not unfrequently have been known to do, by forcing the longer diameter of the wrist across the shorter diameter of the manacle.

The instruments should be of the best workmanship and polish, made so as to be locked by one key throughout, of which a duplicate should be hung up in each restraint room, to enable the House-Surgeon, the Visitor, or any of the Governors, to ascertain at any time the state of the locks. The costly wristlocks made to resist the file, are of course unnecessary here.

Number of Patients—Males 40, Females 18.

(Signed)   GEO. MARR, [Visitor.]

August 18.—The Visitor's Report being read :—Ordered, That the Furnishing Committee do take measures for procuring improved wristlocks for day and night use.

September 8.—Ordered, That glazed Doors be placed at the lower ends of the two Male South Galleries, and the *lower* doors removed at the *North-end* of the North Gallery.

Extract from the House Visitor's Report.

December 22.—I have observed this week, that the House-Porter's valuable time has been occupied in waiting at table, which I consider contrary to the intention of the Governors, in his appointment, and I recommend that this office be performed as heretofore by the house maid.

(Signed)   GEO. MARR, [Visitor.]

Resolved, That the recommendation of the Weekly Visitor respecting the House-Porter, be adopted: that the occupation of the House-Porter be confined as much as possible to the duties for which he was engaged, viz. to relieve the keepers entirely from all employments unconnected with the care of the patients.

December 29.—Ordered, That one pair of night shoes [quarter boots of ticking] for Male patients, and two pairs for Females, be procured.

1835, *January* 14.—Ordered, That the Weekly Board do take measures for completing the Pervision of the galleries, [by means of Sash Doors.]

Ordered, That the Building Committee be requested to consider arrangements for a Sleeping Room, to contain such [Male] patients as may be subject to danger in the night, with accommodation for an attendant to sleep therein.

February 16.—Ordered, That an advance in money be made to the Household in lieu of Beer, at the rate of five pounds a year to Males, and two pounds ten shillings a year to the Females.

Extract from the House Visitor's Report.

1835, *March* 23.—It is very gratifying to see this Institution rising in the public estimation, and more so to observe that there is every prospect of its maintaining the character it has acquired. When the new dormitories become fit for habitation, the sitting rooms for the Male patients will I hope no longer have beds in them; and I wish there was a more immediate prospect of similar accommodation being afforded on the Female side of the house. At present there seems to be more than ordinary attendance required for the Females; but I doubt whether an additional Nurse would not be a great improvement under any circumstances. I beg to suggest to the Governors the expediency of engaging three Nurses instead of two. In that case one of the three might be the constant channel of communication between the Galleries and the body of the House, so that the Galleries would not be left with only one Nurse to attend all the patients during the necessary absence of one for domestic purposes. I am glad to find that it has been determined to make an allowance in money to the household, instead of giving them Beer.

(Signed)   R. PRETYMAN, [Visitor.]

Extracts from the Eleventh Annual Report.

1835, *April.*—By the introduction of Sash Doors throughout the whole of the galleries, the cheerfulness of their appearance has been remarkably increased; while the conduct of the Attendants, and their demeanour towards those under their care, can be readily observed at all times. Frequent observation, the principal duty of the House-Surgeon (disengaged for the purpose from the offices of Secretary and Accountant,) will be greatly facilitated: and the Governors will be enabled to feel entire confidence in the proper treatment of the patients. The opportunities of neglect and harshness behind close and closed doors amidst incompetent witnesses, must be so unlimited, that every obstruction of observation may be considered as an exposure of these institutions to the risk of such consequences.

The best effects have been found to follow the discontinuance of Fermented drink by the patients: and the disturbances formerly not uncommon after dinner, have now disappeared.—To give additional motives for sobriety (a deviation from which is never overlooked by the Board) a pecuniary allowance has been made to all members of the establishment in lieu of malt liquor.

A further review of the instruments of restraint has reduced them to four simple methods :—viz.

Day, 1.—The wrists secured by a flexible connection with a belt round the waist.

2.—The ancles secured by a flexible connection with each other, so as to allow of walking exercise.

Night, 3.—One or both wrists attached by a flexible connection to the side of the bed.

4.—The feet placed in night-shoes, similarly attached to the foot of the bed.

Both the precautions together are very seldom required in the same case, either by day or by night: Strong dresses which cannot readily be torn, and List shoes, generally superseding the necessity of any restraint even in excited cases. The object of restraint is not punishment but security. Every instrument which could confine the fingers themselves has been entirely discarded, for reasons founded upon a distinction between restraints which render a patient harmless, and those which would render him unable to employ the remains of his reason to assist himself on proper occasions. The present suffering and future ill consequences resulting from the neglect of this distinction, have been forcibly depicted in the evidence* given by Mr. John Haslam,

---

* QUESTION.—How are the hands secured [in Bethlem]? With chains?

ANSWER.—A manacle is a means of confining the wrists, leaving the fingers at liberty, but rendering them incapable of separating their arms for the purposes of effecting violence.

Q.—Might not violence be effected by both the hands?

A.—No, you cannot be afraid of any man so secured.

Apothecary for more than twenty years at Bethlem, during an examination upon this subject before a Committee of the House of Commons.—The number of instances of restraint has continued further to diminish in a striking manner, as will appear by an abstract from the Report of the Weekly

Q.—You think that the hands so secured with irons, is less objectionable than when secured by a strait-waistcoat? A.—A thousand times.

Q.—Can the patient move his hands to his face?

A.—Certainly; it is merely a security round each wrist.

Q.—Is he not capable of doing himself an injury with his hands secured in that way?

A.—No; he is not able to strangle himself, or to fix the apparatus to hang himself, or do any injury to himself, or any body else.

Q.—Is he not capable of striking another person with his hands secured with irons?

A.—The hands put up even of a timid person would prevent it.

Q.—Is he not capable of striking at another person that may come in his way? A.—Not to hurt him; he can strike him, but not to hurt him.

Q.—Then it is your opinion, if a man is handcuffed in the manner already described, a man of common bodily strength, such as is fit to be employed as a keeper, need not be afraid of injury from the most outrageous Maniac?

A.—As far as the hands are concerned, certainly not.

Q.—If his legs or feet were confined in the usual manner by footlocks?

A.—Then he would be an innoxious animal.

Q.—What are the disadvantages you conceive attending on the use of a strait-waistcoat?

A.—The hands are completely confined; if the strait-waistcoat be tied tightly, respiration is prevented or impeded, and it is always at the mercy of the keeper how tight he chooses to tie the waistcoat. If the patient be irritated by itching in any part, he is unable to administer the relief by scratching, or if troubled with flies; in hot weather it is a painful incumbrance, and if not changed is liable to absorb a great deal of perspiration, which renders sometimes the skin excoriated. He cannot wipe his nose, and he becomes a driveller in consequence; he cannot assist himself on natural occasions, or possess personal cleanliness as long as the strait-waistcoat is applied. Then there is another very curious effect that has resulted from keeping on the strait-waistcoat for a considerable time; the nails are pinched up, and I have seen some instances where patients have been long kept in the strait-waistcoat, where the nail has resembled the claw of an animal; so that I can pretty nearly judge by the look of the hand of a lunatic, if I do not see his face, whether he has been the subject of a strait-waistcoat a long while.

Visitor, *August* 10, 1834, who observes " That he has much gratification in being able to state that not a single male patient has been under restraint since the 16th day of July, and not one female patient since the 1st of August," up to the above date.

(Signed) T. MANNERS SUTTON,

Chairman.

April 20.—Ordered, That the person of every Patient [while bathing] be examined especially and carefully by the House-Surgeon and Matron respectively; and that marks (if any) found upon their persons, be reported in the " Weekly Memorandum Book," forthwith to the Board.

1835, *July* 6.—Ordered, That whenever it may become absolutely necessary to overpower a Refractory Patient, two attendants be employed for that purpose, to prevent as much as possible the risk of resistance and struggle.

Extract from the " Governors' Memorandum Book."

July 8.—We, the Undersigned, present at the Quarterly Board this day, having inspected the Asylum, report that we found every part of the Establishment clean and orderly. We cannot avoid expressing our high approbation on noticing the complete opportunity now afforded to the Officers and Governors of observing the conduct of the Attendants towards the patients through the sash doors, which pervade the whole of the galleries.——

(Signed) THOS. BRAILSFORD,

W. M. PIERCE,

W. B. R. BURTON.

July 8.—Resolved, That this Board in acknowledging the services of Mr. Hadwen, during the period of fifteen months that he held the situation of House-Surgeon of this Institution, feel called upon to express their high approbation of the very small proportion of instances of Restraint, which have occurred amongst the Patients under his care.

House Visitor's Report.

1835, *August* 17.—I have visited the Asylum regularly the last week, and am satisfied that every attention is paid to the health and comfort of the Patients. Mr. Hill informs me it has not been necessary to put any of them under Restraint for the ten last days. The wards of every part of the building are perfectly clean, and the provisions very good.

Patients—Males 37, Females 20.

(Signed)   G. T. PRETYMAN, [Visitor.]

Extract from the House Visitor's Report.

September 7.—I have much satisfaction in stating we have not had one Patient under restraint or confinement since the 14th of last August.

Number of Patients—Males 39, Females 20.

(Signed)   JOHN WM. STURGES, [Visitor.]

September 14.—Ordered, That a third Nurse be engaged, so that neither of the galleries may be left unattended at any time, and the patients may have an opportunity of walking out occasionally into the country.

[*Extract from the Revised Regulations.*]
1835, *October* 14.

That strong dresses of Barragon or Sacking be procured for the Patients who tear their clothes, to prevent the necessity of Restraints.

House Visitor's Report.

1836, *Jan.* 18.—I have great pleasure in reporting my entire approbation of the manner in which every department of this Institution is conducted ; and in observing the many and important improvements which have been made since my last visit. The regularity and order which prevail in the domestic economy of the house is exceedingly creditable to all ; but the visible alteration which has taken place in the state of the Patients, in the comforts which are afforded to them, and in their capability of enjoying those comforts, must be peculiarly gratifying to those who take an interest in the management and in the character of the Institution. Restraints upon the person of the patients have been for some time gradually diminished in number, and this last week has by no means been the only one lately in which not a single patient has been put under any restraint whatever. On referring to the Minute Book, I observe that stockings were produced to the Board on the 30th of November last, knitted by female patients, and last week some nightcaps were produced also from the same source ; and such employment must be a striking evidence of that general quiet and of that mild and innocent character of confinement, which some years ago would never have been believed safe or even possible in a Lunatic Asylum.

The fitting up of one large room at the end of the Dormitory with several beds in it for the melancholy patients, is a new feature in this Institution ; but although a Keeper is occupying the adjoining cell, I shall never think that all possible precautions are taken against the commission of suicide, or of other acts of violence in the night, until a regular night-watch is established in the house. Patients are now left for many hours alone, and much mischief might be done though a Keeper were sleeping in the very next apartment ; I therefore beg to recommend to the Governors that some arrangement should be immediately made by which the house should never be suffered to be left without a regular watchman, and I conceive this duty might be performed by the Keepers now

in the House. Another reason for my earnest recommendation of this arrangement is that it would render unnecessary
the division of the new Dormitory into another range of cells.
No inconvenience has arisen from the placing several beds in
one room, nor can I see any objection to the converting the
Dormitory as it now is, into an open ward by the simple introduction of beds; it rather seems desirable to preserve the
handsome appearance of that new Gallery, which would be
totally lost by the erection of the proposed partition walls.

I must confess I am now anxious to see a day room built
for the North Gallery, and some accommodation afforded to
the Female patients, who are far from enjoying their share of
the comforts and advantages of Classification. If the Watch
should be established, and if the money wanted for the new
partition walls in the Dormitory, should thus be saved, perhaps it would be practicable to proceed directly with these
desirable improvements, which more immediately concern the
comfort of the patients, and which have been long contem-
plated.

[Number of Patients—Males 42, Females 22.]

(*Signed*)   R. Pretyman, [Visitor.]

1836, *January* 25.—The Report of the Weekly Visitor
having been read, it was resolved that a Night Watch be
established in the new Upper Gallery and Dormitory; and
the four male attendants having undertaken it, that they be
allowed an addition of five pounds each to their yearly
wages.

That beds be procured to be placed in the new Upper
Gallery as in an open ward, and that no partitions be put up
therein.

Extract from the House Visitor's Report.

March 7.—I have much pleasure in observing, that
although there are at the present time 74 Patients in the

House, not one has any instrument of restraint on, nor has there been any used for the three last months, which is a sufficient proof that the Keepers and Nurses are active and vigilant in their duty and attentive to their Patients, and reflects also much credit upon the Director, whose unremitting attention to the important duties of his office I have much pleasure in noticing.

Number of Patients—Males 48, Females 26.

(Signed,) JOHN FARDELL, [Visitor.]

Extracts from the Twelfth Annual Report.

1836, *March* 21.—The additional Building over the North Gallery, mentioned in the Report of the preceding year, is now finished and in occupation. One part of it has been partitioned off into single Sleeping-rooms, and the other part appropriated as a Dormitory under Night Watch,* for [Male] Patients disposed to injure themselves, or otherwise requiring special vigilance.

In consequence of the crowded state of the Female side of the house, and the want of proper means of Classification, the Boards found a necessity for discharging some incurable Female Patients,[†] who were particularly troublesome and annoying to the remainder. An order has since been made for commencing a Gallery for the Insensible Class of Female Patients, corresponding with that on the Male side; the order has been limited in its extent by the state of the disposable funds, which will not admit of more than a small advance in this building at present.

Notwithstanding the increased number of Patients, (now 74,) the Boards have observed with much satisfaction, that

---

* The Attendant wears list shoes to prevent disturbing the Patients; matting is laid down for him to walk upon; a dull light is allowed.

[† Not any patient has been either refused admission or discharged on such account, since the date of my appointment in July, 1835. R. G. Hill.]

the amount of Instances of Restraint has continued rapidly to diminish. There is no doubt that

The complete means of Classification afforded by the improved Construction of the Building—

The Dormitory under Night Watch—

The ample sufficiency of Attendants of good temper and sufficient bodily power—

Their Non-occupation in any other duty than the personal care of the Patients—

The Practice of this duty secured by the introduction of Sash Doors throughout the House—

The wholesome manner in which the Public eye is brought to bear upon the treatment of the Patients—

The separate Depository for the Instruments of Restraint—

The Official authority required for each instance of their application, and the subsequent Registry—

The use of Strong Dresses for Patients who would tear their clothes :—and of List Shoes for those disposed to do injury with their feet—

The cheerful aspect of the Apartments, Grounds, and Prospects—

The abundant Exercise in the open air—

The encouragement of Employments, Sports, and Amusements—

The total Abstinence from Fermented Liquors—

have each contributed to this effect. Still more however must always depend upon the *personal* attention of the House-Surgeon to the Patients, and upon his insisting and actually seeing, (for in no other way can he know) that they habitually receive the same care from the Attendants; whose inclination, it must be remembered, would naturally lead them to the confinement of the Patients to save themselves from trouble.

Three successive months (excepting one day) have now elapsed without the occurrence of a single instance of Restraint in this establishment : and out of thirty-six weeks that the House-Surgeon has held his present situation, twenty-five whole weeks (excepting two days) have been passed without any recourse to such means, and even without an instance of confinement to a separate room.

(Signed) R. Pretyman, Chairman.

August 1.——Ordered, That in consequence of the very diminished use of instruments of Restraint since the completion of the arrangements on the Male side of the House, the number of instruments be reduced to four [sizes] of each sort, and that the remainder be disposed of.

October 12.——Resolved, That it is highly expedient to take immediate measures for erecting a Female Insensible Gallery, and that the Weekly Board be empowered to proceed accordingly.

That the Very Reverend the Dean, the Treasurer, Sir E. Ff. Bromhead, Bart., and the Physicians be a Committee to prepare a Circular for aid in the above object, addressed to the principal Proprietors of the County, who have not already contributed to the funds of the Institution.

November 14.——Ordered, That Sash Doors be continued throughout the whole of the Day Apartments.

December 5.——Resolved, on a representation from the House-Surgeon, That the Female attendants be not employed in sewing, which prevents them from paying the necessary attention to the patients.

Extracts from the Thirteenth Annual Report.

1837. *April* 12.——It cannot be too widely made known that in a properly constructed and well regulated Asylum, the Insane may be treated not only much more easily and effectually, but also much more mildly than at their own home, where the unadapted arrangements of the Dwelling and Grounds, and the presence of Relatives and Dependants, oppose unceasing impediments to Recovery, and often produce an aggravation of the complaint by the restraint and close confinement which may become unavoidable under the circumstances.*

The present House Surgeon has expressed his own belief, founded on experience in this house, that it may be possible to conduct an Institution for the Insane without having recourse to the employment of any instruments of Restraint whatsoever. He has certainly made a striking advance towards verifying this opinion, by conducting the Male, (the completed) side of the house, with but a solitary instance of such restraint, either by day or by night, during the course of the sixteen last months, and that applied only for about six hours, during his absence; nor is it impossible, when the Buildings can be finished, that an example may be offered of an Asylum, in which undivided personal attention towards the Patients shall be altogether substituted for the use of Instruments.†

---

* Patients are frequently brought to this Asylum under distressing Restraints, which have been kept constantly applied for several weeks or months together, and in one instance for more than twenty years. At the Bicêtre in Paris, the chains imposed at the time of admission were not ever removed till death : the humane and intelligent Pinel, after an arduous struggle with the authorities, succeeded at last in breaking through this barbarous custom, and restored the inmates to ease, comfort, and recovery.

† Soon after the date of a Regulation made in this house (February, 1829) requiring that one of the Attendants should sit up with any Patient confined in a Strait-waistcoat during the night, the use of that Instrument, previously considered indispensible, *totally* disappeared : even the slight trouble of entering the fact of any Restraint was found in the same manner to produce a diminution. Whenever for any reason, Patients are locked up from the rest in the day time, a ticket denoting the circumstance should be hung upon each door; otherwise under the greatest appearance of frankness and openness to inspection, Patients

By the degree of approach to this Result of sound Construction, of Management, and of Official Conduct, ought the excellence of every Public Asylum to be tested. The Governors must not allow their attention to be seduced from this point by the bustle and glare of any operations,* which may give occasional Employment to a portion of the Inmates, (as in Husbandry, the Management of Cattle, &c., &c.,) and yet pass over the least sensible and the most helpless, and create an erroneous impression relative to the general treatment of the Patients. Such operations moreover afford pleas for extravagant expenditure and costly establishment,† disguised amidst multiplied concerns and complicated accounts, often even under delusive appearances of economy or profit. Ample means of quiet engagement in the *open air* (an essential to Recovery) may be provided without investments of Capital, or special Superintendance, and without creating Dependants upon the house, or multiplying the avocations of the Officer upon whose vigilant supervision and minute personal attention to the condition of each individual Patient, the comfort, health, and mental improvement of the whole must depend.

may be suffering all the miseries of confinement and neglect, unseen and unsuspected by the Visitor.

* See the Tenth Report of this Institution.

† A costly and luxurious scale in the Household of any Public Charity, if suffered to grow up through a want of firmness on the part of the Boards, will produce inevitably a laxity of discipline throughout the house. It necessarily begets indolence, and leads throughout the establishment to the evasion of troublesome duties—to severity as the readiest means of control—to habitual confinement as the safeguard against occasional violence or escape—to injured health and loathsome habits, induced by confining the fingers with " Muffs," " Sleeves," " Gloves," and other cruel inventions—to revolting substitutes for the attention due to Insensible Patients—to entertaining strangers in the house, with its train of mischievous consequences—and to the perpetuation of misrule by discountenancing, under a pretext of injury to the Patients, such wholesome and efficient public inspection, as might expose and rectify abuse.

Sedentary Employments, such as Manufactures, Handicrafts, &c., cannot be considered in themselves generally friendly to health; and if admissible at all into an Asylum, require caution and strict vigilant Regulation. The sedentary habits required by such employments are also unquestionably injurious to the free action of the alimentary canal, which must be considered an object of primary attention in mental disorder; nor can we find, except in very large Establishments, a number of Patients suitable for carrying into effect the particular manufactures which may be introduced. Any quiet engagements (such as knitting, &c.) which can be conducted without the expense of building work-rooms for the purpose, or purchasing and maintaining machinery, or requiring special superintendance, or interfering with the ordinary duties of the usual attendants, or demanding a stooping posture, or introducing dangerous implements,—and which can be always at hand, and adopted by the Patients individually, while standing or sitting or walking, either within doors, or in the open air,—are particularly adapted for the use of the Insane, whose irregular capacity for employment, and whose capricious inclinations usually unfit them for settled attention and steady application. Extraordinary bodily exertion under *any* employment, never ought to be encouraged, more especially by stimulating indulgences in fermented liquors or narcotic drugs; nor should any emolument or advantage whatsoever be derived by members of the Establishment; nor ought the convenience arising from the skill or usefulness of any Patient, to be a motive for protracting his stay.

A decidedly improved health has been found to follow the total disuse of fermented liquor, and the more generous diet which has been substituted. The true causes of mortality, especially in establishments which admit the poor, may be traced to the depressing effects of damp, cold, and low diet; the previous operation of these may show itself after admission, even in well conducted establishments.

(Signed)   W. M. PIERCE, Chairman.

May 8.—Ordered, That occasional assistance be hired to help and superintend the Patients employed in casual labour.

May 15.—Ordered, That whenever any Patient may be locked up apart from the rest, a ticket noting the circumstance be hung upon the door.

July 12.—At a General Quarterly Board, &c.

The following minute of the Weekly Board of Governors holden June, 26, 1837, being read,

> Ordered, That special notice be given that it is intended at the next General Quarterly Board of Governors of the Lincoln Lunatic Asylum, to take into consideration the best means of raising on the security of the Property, sufficient funds for the completion of the Buildings and the purchase of certain Land adjoining the Asylum grounds, required for the purposes thereof.

Resolved, That this Board approves and confirms the matter of the above minute.

Resolved and ordered, That the sum of £2000. be raised on Mortgage, or Deposit of the Deeds, &c., &c.

Extracts from the House Visitor's Report.

September 11.—I visited the Asylum during the past week. On my first visit the Female patients were in a frightfully excited and disturbed state: the Men were much more tranquil. I am glad to find that progress is making in the new works of the north-west ward, [for Insensible Females,] and would urge upon the Board the necessity of its early completion. The indiscriminate association of the noisy and disturbed patients, with those enjoying sane intervals, and desirous of repose and quiet, must be very distressing to the latter, and materially interfere with their chances of recovery.

[Number of Patients—Males 61, Females 38.]

(*Signed*) R. Mason, [Visitor.]

October 2.—Ordered, That the Chairs used formerly for the double purpose of Night Chairs and of Restraint, [long fallen into disuse,] be worked up.

October 11.—Resolved, That this Board is highly sensible of the House-Surgeon's* successful exertions in reducing the number of Restraints, and his readiness on every occasion to undertake any trouble for the benefit of the Institution, and that it be recommended to the Weekly Board to reconsider the amount of his salary.

December 4.—Resolved, That a Night-watch be established on the Female side of the House, and a Nurse engaged.

Fourteenth Annual Report.

1838, *March.*—At the General Board in July last, the Governors having taken into consideration the pressing inconveniences, arising from the inadequate accommodation, and the unfinished state of the Female side of the Asylum, as described in the preceding Annual Report, resolved upon applying to the Lincoln Bank for a credit of £2000. on deposit of the writings of the Trust Estate. This application was readily acceded to, and considerable progress has been made in carrying into effect the objects of the loan, under the very economical management of Mr. Hartley, whose professional ability as Surveyor of this Establishment is well known. A large accession of room has thus been obtained

* Mr. R. G. Hill.

for the reception and necessary Classification of Female patients, and a long desired purchase has been effected of about an acre of ground, immediately adjoining the Female portion of the Building. All the more Sensible of either sex will now be enabled to enjoy the invaluable privilege of taking exercise in the open air, without interruption, in ample space, and with cheerful distant scenery, during any part of the day whenever the weather will permit : and the former Airing Courts of this Class of the Patients may be applied to the enlargement of the remainder, so as to gain for the less Sensible Class, much healthful and convenient room, long seriously needed under their increase of numbers.

The Boards have to acknowledge with gratitude numerous liberal donations in aid of the above objects, from parties whose names are recorded in the annexed list of Benefactors. The situation well merits every exertion which can be made to enhance the natural advantages. A late writer thus describes it. *" The Asylum is built on the prominent south-" western brow of the lofty hill which forms the scite of the " Castle, and consequently commands one of the finest pro-" spects in the County. The City lies partly to the east, " and partly below the hill towards the south-east, so situated " as neither by smoke nor business to become any annoyance " to the inmates of the Asylum. On the west and south-" west is an extensive plain, once covered with water, but " now completely drained ; the nearer part a large open " common field, in which is the race-ground, and a great " part of that ancient canal, the Fossdyke. Beyond, a fine " cultivated Country, interspersed with woods, seats, and " spires, of an extent truly astonishing, and only bounded by " the high grounds of Leicestershire and Nottinghamshire, " and the towering mountains of the Peak. Thus elevated " in its situation, open to the western breezes, and sheltered

* The Lincolnshire Cabinet.

" from the cutting north and north-west winds, it enjoys an
" air, pure and salubrious, unimpregnated by miasma, un-
" contaminated by the effluvia of a crowded population."

There is now an increased confidence that the anticipations of the last year may be fulfilled, and that "An example
" may be offered of a Public Asylum, in which undivided
" personal attention towards the Patients shall be altogether
" substituted for the use of Instruments of Restraint." The
bold conception of pushing the mitigation of restraint to the
extent of actually and formally abolishing the practice,
mentioned in the last Report as due to Mr. Hill the House-
Surgeon, seems to be justified by the following abstract of a
statistical Table,* showing the rapid advance of the abatement of restraints in this Asylum, under an improved Construction of the Building, Night-watching, and attentive
Supervision. We may venture to affirm, that this is the
first frank statement of the common practice of restraints,
hitherto laid before a British Public. (See Table in the
Appendix C.)

This striking progress of amelioration affords great encouragement for persevering in a system so successfully
commenced ; and the more so, as a corresponding decrease
of violence, accidents, and revolting habits, has accompanied
the change. Under any system whatsoever, violence must be
expected occasionally to exhibit itself, and produce its effects
in a Lunatic Asylum ; but the comparative rarity of such
collisions in this Asylum since the alteration of the Building,
the discontinuance of fermented drink, and an habitual
presence of attendants in lieu of restraints, has shown that
coercion may be safely dispensed with. On the same prin-

---

* This Table was prepared by Mr. Hill, who since his appointment in July,
1835, has, on this, as well as every other occasion, faithfully and unsparingly
exerted himself to serve the interests of the Institution. It is in the power of an
unwilling officer to make any improvements fail in practice.

ciple it has been observed, that the number of escapes and outrages in prisons has materially diminished since the time that the legislature forbade the ordinary use of irons. There is little doubt that the constraint upon free motion, so commonly employed in violation of a relief called for and indicated by nature under a redundant excitability, must be as distressing and injurious to the Insane, as would be a systematic suppression of the noisy mobility of Childhood. The mischievous ingenuity sometimes exhibited in Instruments of Restraint, tends to mislead the feelings of the public, who ought to keep steadily in view that, without any exception, *every* invention (such as the Chair of restraint, &c.) must impede motion and the proper action of the system, must irritate the Patient, encourage loathsome habits, and discourage all tendency to self control. The very principle of such bodily coercion is unsound and unphilosophical.

The erroneous prepossessions of society on the subject of Insanity, often lead strangers, while unconsciously surrounded by all the worst cases in this Asylum, to enquire where are the furious and violent; and some strangers can with difficulty be induced to believe, that the unoffending peaceful persons amidst whom they are standing, are the very objects of their inquiry and alarm, subjected to no other control than the habitual presence of steady, watchful, and powerful attendants. The popular belief in the ungovernable ferocity of the Insane, encouraged by persons more studious of their own ease and enjoyment than that of the Patients intrusted to their care, has been very mischievous, and has tended to excuse restraints and other severities, on the assumption of their necessity; whereas in truth it is this very practice which renders the complaint intractable, and gives to it a character of exacerbation seeming to justify both the prejudice and the treatment. Such prejudices and their consequences can only be corrected, by opening examples of a milder management to the inspection of Society, which has a deep personal concern in the mild or harsh treatment of a complaint, which may affect *any*, either personally or through relatives and friends.

During the period when restraints were so freely resorted to in this and other Asylums, it could be little imagined by strangers permitted to see the condition of only a selected portion of the Patients, exercising or engaged in the beautiful Fore-grounds, or in some of the cheerful Galleries in front—that behind this scene were lingering under restraint such a large proportion of the Patients. The Public has generally seen what it is least important that they should see. Dr. Farre observes, The words of the talented Samuel Tuke on this subject are golden : " *I believe that I am not too* " *sanguine when I say, that for one evil arising from accidental* " *Visitation, ninety-nine will be prevented. The evils of Visit-* " *ation are speculative bugbears, to which practical men have* " *too often found it convenient to give the character of reality.*"

The Dietary of the Third Rank Patients has received an addition of animal food, which is now allowed daily instead of for four days only in the week as heretofore. A corresponding diminution in the consumption of farinaceous food, and the entire disuse of fermented drink (by reason of its stimulating property,) have obviated the necessity of any increased charge on this account; while the improved digestible and nutritious quality of the food, will render it more suitable for the impaired nervous condition of the Patients. A recent Parliamentary inquiry has elicited the fact, that a high rate of mortality in Asylums for the Insane, usually accompanies a low rate of charge; the latter of course implying inferiority of diet, and warmth, and attendance, as the chief sources of reduced cost.

Statistical observations have determined that Insanity tends to accelerate the rate of mortality: how much of this consequence may justly be attributed to the complaint, and its usual accompaniment of latent or open organic disease, and how much to improper treatment, remains yet to be ascertained. It is probable that as the number of public Lunatic Asylums shall continue to increase, the treatment of the Insane will continue to improve by comparison of practice: provided that the size of the Establishments be kept within such limits, as not to place the management beyond the control of the Boards, nor out of the reach of minute inspection* in every department, nor beyond the possibility of particular professional attention being paid to the case of each individual Patient. Under such circumstances the Statistics of future years may show results more favourable than those of the past, which embrace a period when public Lunatic Asylums were comparatively few, and under a revolting system.

(Signed)   E. P. CHARLESWORTH,

Chairman.

1838, *April* 2.—Ordered, That an additional male and an additional female attendant be engaged, at the request of the House-Surgeon, as entered in the " Board Memorandum Book."

That a Strait-waistcoat and a Leathern Muff found by the Matron in the linen cupboard, be removed from the stock of the Institution.

Physician's Report.

April 18.—The House-Surgeon informs me that out of twenty-nine patients who have been brought [to the Asylum] since the time of his appointment, *insensible to the calls of nature*, from the previous use of the strait-waistcoat, nineteen have been restored to habits of cleanliness.

(Signed)   E. P. CHARLESWORTH,

[Attending Physician.]

Physician's Report.

June 3.—In the short space of time since I left ——
yesterday raving and blaspheming, and disposed to injure
those about her, if she had been left unwatched, she has
become quiet and tractable, having been subjected only to
close and careful observation from the Attendants, and to
no other description of restraint nor to seclusion.

(*Signed*)　　　E. P. CHARLESWORTH,
　　　　　　　　　　[Attending Physician.]

Extract from the House Visitor's Report.

July 2.—I was glad to find the new wing for [Insensible]
Female patients in use; the advantages of it are already
manifest in the improved state of that Class of inmates..

[Number of Patients—Males 55, Females 42.]

(*Signed*)　　　R. MASON, [Visitor.]

July 11.—Resolved, That the thanks of this Board be
given to the House-Surgeon for a series of Statistical Tables
presented by him, shewing the instances and amount of the
Restraints employed in this Establishment since the commencement of their Registry in 1829; with various other
valuable extracts from the documents of the Institution.

Physician's Report.

July 31.—I have observed with much satisfaction, the
wholesome and agreeable influence upon the patients, of the
fires kept up in their sitting rooms during a great part of the
present month of July, which has been unusually cold. The
languid state of the circulation of the generality of Lunatics,
and their indisposition towards active movement, conspire
to keep the temperature of their bodies below the natural
and healthy standard; and render an extraordinary supply
of artificial warmth especially necessary for them.

The striking quietness, gentleness, and docility of the inmates of this Institution, may not unreasonably be attributed to the extraordinary attention paid to their comforts, and the care taken to preserve them from causes of annoyance and irritation. In proof of this may be quoted the peaceable and placid demeanour of the Female patients in their roomy new north Gallery, as compared with their previous violent and restless demeanour when crowded together in their former small apartment.

(Signed)   E. P. CHARLESWORTH,

[Attending Physician.]

September 17.—Ordered, That all Instruments of Restraint used by the friends of Patients for bringing them to the Asylum, be always returned at the time.

September 24.—Ordered, That no Officer, Attendant, or Servant keep in his private possession on the premises any Instruments of Restraint.

B.

A

TABULAR VIEW

OF THE

SEVERAL INSTANCES

OF

RESTRAINT, COERCION, AND SECLUSION,

USED IN THE

LINCOLN LUNATIC ASYLUM,

FROM MARCH 16TH, 1829, TO MARCH 22ND, 1837,

WHEN THE PRACTICE WAS WHOLLY DISCONTINUED.

C.

SUMMARY OF THE PRECEDING TABLES.

Year.	Total number of Patients in the House.	Total number of Patients Restrained.	Total number of Instances of Restraint.	Total number of Hours passed under Restraint.
1829*	72	39	1727	20,424
1830	92	54	2364	27,113¼
1831	70	40	1004	10,830
1832	81	55	1401	15,671½
1833	87	44	1109	12,003½
1834	109	45	647	6,597
1835	108	28	323	2,874
1836	115	12	39	334
1837	130	2	3	28

After deducting the number of Patients introduced in the above Table more than once in the years 1829-30-31-32-33-34-35, and also the re-admitted cases within the same period, the actual number of Patients restrained in the course of such seven years was, 169 :—

Of these 169, there remained in the House at the end of such seven years, 43 :—

Of these remaining 43, there were discharged from the Books during the years 1836-7, *not having been restrained at all* during any part of such two years 11

————————————— having been restrained only for about *seven hours* during any part of such two years ... 2

———— remained in the House December 31, 1837, *not having been restrained at all* during any part of such two years 29

————————————— having been restrained *once only* (for about nine hours) during any part of such two years ... 1

————

43

————

From March 16th.

D.

NUMBER OF SUICIDES

AND

THEIR APPARENT CONNEXION WITH RESTRAINTS.

Date of House-Surgeon's Appointment.	Period Included.	Number of Patients Treated.	Number of Suicides.	Proportion of Suicides.	Rate of Coercion.
April 26, 1820.	10½ years	334	2	1 in 167	Maximum
October 14, 1830.	3½ years } 4¾ years	173 } 242*	2 } 5	1 in 86½ } 1 in 48½	Medium
April 9, 1834.	1¼ year	120	3	1 in 40	
July 8, 1835.	3¼ years	246	0	0 in 246	Minimum

* From this Total 51 have been deducted, being the number left in the House at the time of the third House-Surgeon's appointment, and therefore necessarily counted as under treatment both of himself and his predecessor.

E.

STATISTICAL TABLES

OF THE

LINCOLN LUNATIC ASYLUM.

The Tables marked thus * are from the Annual Statements of the Institution.

*TABLE I.

Number of the Patients Admitted, and of those Discharged from the Books,

From April 26, 1820, to December 31, 1828.

	M.	F.	Tot.
Admitted	136	99	235
Re-admitted cases	11	10	21
Discharged	122	92	214
Remained December 31, 1828	25	17	42

*TABLE II.

State of the Patients when Discharged from the Books,

From April 26, 1820, to December 31, 1828.

Recovered	102
Improved	34
Removed during treatment	39
Improper object	1
By order of the Board	1
Escaped	0
Dead	37

*TABLE III.

Causes of the Deaths,

From April 26, 1820, to December 31, 1828.

Apoplexy	3	Gradual Exhaustion	8
Catalepsy	1	Inflammation of the Brain	1
Dropsy	6	Locked Jaw	1
Dying when admitted	4	Maniacal Exhaustion	1
Epilepsy	4	Old Age	3
Fever	1	Psoas Abscess	1
Found dead in bed	1	Suicide	2

TABLE IV.

Modes of Self-destruction, with Dates and Patients' Nos.

1821—August   27 .... No. 28 .... Hanging.
1824—November 15 .... No. 107 .... Hanging.

1829.

*TABLE V.

Number of the Patients Admitted, and of those Discharged from the Books,

From January 1, 1829, to December 31, 1829.

	M.	F.	Tot.
Remained January 1, 1829	25	17	42
Admitted in 1829	24	12	36
Re-admitted in 1829	5	0	5
Discharged in 1829	18	16	34
Remaining December 31, 1829	36	13	49

*TABLE VI.

State of the Patients when Discharged from the Books,
From January 1, 1829, to December 31, 1829.

Recovered.. 22
Improved 5
Removed during treatment...................................... 6
Improper object 0
By order of the Board.. 0
Escaped 0
Dead 1

*TABLE VII.

Cause of the Death in 1829.
Maniacal Exhaustion.

1830.

----

*TABLE VIII.

Number of the Patients Admitted, and of those Discharged from the Books,
From January 1, 1830, to December 31, 1830.

	M.	F.	Tot.
Remained January 1, 1830.........	36	13	49
Admitted in 1830	17	13	30
Re-admitted in 1830	8	5	13
Discharged in 1830..............	33	18	51
Remaining December 31, 1830	28	13	41

*TABLE IX.

State of the Patients when Discharged from the Books,
From January 1, 1830, to December 31, 1830.

Recovered.. 29
Improved 4
Removed during treatment...................................... 9
Improper object 0
By order of the Board.. 0
Escaped 1
Dead 8

*TABLE X.

Causes of the Deaths in 1830.

Epilepsy .... 1 | Gradual Exhaustion 6
Paralysis 1

1831.

---

*TABLE XI.

Number of the Patients Admitted, and of those Discharged from the Books,
From January 1, 1831, to December 31, 1831.

	M.	F.	Tot.
Remained January 1, 1831	28	13	41
Admitted in 1831	13	7	20
Re-admitted in 1831	3	6	9
Discharged in 1831	13	13	26
Remaining December 31, 1831	31	13	44

*TABLE XII.

State of the Patients when Discharged from the Books,

From January 1, 1831, to December 31, 1831.

Recovered	11
Improved	1
Removed during treatment	5
Improper object	0
By order of the Board	0
Escaped	0
Dead	9

*TABLE XIII.

Causes of the Deaths in 1831.

Epilepsy	2	Gradual Exhaustion	5
Fever	1	Suicide	1

TABLE XIV.

Mode of Self-destruction, with Date and Patient's No.

May 18 .... No. 343 .... Hanging.

1832.

*TABLE XV.

Number of the Patients Admitted, and of those Discharged from the Books,

From January 1, 1832, to December 31, 1832.

	M.	F.	Tot.
Remained January 1, 1832	31	13	44
Admitted in 1832	18	12	30
Re-admitted in 1832	6	1	7
Discharged in 1832	19	15	34
Remaining December 31, 1832	36	11	47

*TABLE XVI.

State of the Patients when Discharged from the Books,
From January 1, 1832, to December 31, 1832.

Recovered 10
Improved 4
Removed during treatment 5
Improper object 0
By order of the Board 2
Escaped 1
Dead 12

*TABLE XVII.

Causes of the Deaths in 1832.

Abscess of the Brain	1	Epilepsy	1
Diarrhœa	3	Gradual Exhaustion	1
Maniacal Exhaustion	2	Tabes	4

1833.

---

*TABLE XVIII.

*Number of the Patients Admitted, and of those Discharged
from the Books,*
From January 1, 1833, to December 31, 1833.

	M.	F.	Tot.
Remained January 1, 1833	36	11	47
Admitted in 1833	17	17	34
Re-admitted in 1833	2	4	6
Discharged in 1833	20	17	37
Remaining December 31, 1833	35	15	50

*TABLE XIX.

State of the Patients when Discharged from the Books,

From January 1, 1833, to December 31, 1833.

Recovered	12
Improved	3
Removed during treatment	10
Improper object	0
By order of the Board	2
Escaped	1
Dead	9

*TABLE XX.

Causes of the Deaths in 1833.

Apoplexy	1	Maniacal Exhaustion	1
Fever	1	Psoas Abscess	1
Gradual Exhaustion	3	Suicide	1
	Tabes	1	

TABLE XXI.

Mode of Self-destruction, with Date and Patient's No.

April 29 .... No. 405 .... Burning.

1834.

*TABLE XXII.

Number of the Patients Admitted, and of those Discharged from the Books,

From January 1, 1834, to December 31, 1834.

	M.	F.	Tot.
Remained January 1, 1834	35	15	50
Admitted in 1834	22	18	40
Re-admitted in 1834	9	10	19
Discharged in 1834	24	19	43
Remaining December 31, 1834	42	24	66

*TABLE XXIII.

State of the Patients when Discharged from the Books,

From January 1, 1834, to December 31, 1834.

Recovered... 17
Improved 5
Removed during treatment...................................... 15
Improper object 0
By order of the Board.. 2
Escaped 0
Dead... 4

*TABLE XXIV.

Causes of the Deaths in 1834.

Dying when admitted ...... 1 | Found dead in bed 1
Suicide 2

TABLE XXV.

Modes of Self-destruction, with Dates and Patients' Nos.

July   5 ... No. 453 ... Strangling.
August 1 ... No. 455 ... Knocking the head against the wall.

---

1 8 3 5 .

*TABLE XXVI.

Number of the Patients Admitted, and of those Discharged from the Books,

From January 1, 1835, to December 31, 1835.

	M.	F.	Tot.
Remained January 1, 1835......................	42	24	66
Admitted in 1835	15	17	32
Re-admitted in 1835	7	3	10
Discharged in 1835.............................	23	23	46
Remaining December 31, 1835	41	21	62

*TABLE XXVII.

State of the Patients when Discharged from the Books,

From January 1, 1835, to December 31, 1835.

Recovered	16
Improved	2
Removed during treatment	13
Improper object	0
By order of the Board	5
Escaped	1
Dead	9

*TABLE XXVIII.

Causes of the Deaths in 1835.

Apoplexy	1	Maniacal Exhaustion	1
Gradual Exhaustion	1	Suicide	1
Inflamed Lungs	2	Ulcerated Bowels	1
Inflamed Parotid Gland	1	Water in the Head	1

TABLE XXIX.

Mode of Self-destruction, with Date and Patient's No.

May 20 .... No. 515 .... Hanging.

*TABLE XXX.

Weekly Return of the State of the Patients.

From June 22 to June 29, 1835.	M.	F.	Totals
Number of Patients in the House	38	21	59
First Rank	3	3	6
Second Rank	4	0	4
Third Rank	31	18	49
Maintained by their Friends	16	7	23
Maintained by the Public	22	14	36
Less than 1 year since the 1st attack ...	8	7	15
More than 1 year since the 1st attack ...	30	14	44
Not expected to recover	30	15	45
Expected to recover	8	6	14
Convalescent	2	3	5
Employed in the last week	no return		
Attended Chapel on Sunday	19	9	28
Cases of Idiotcy	0	1	1
Cases of Epilepsy	3	1	4
Cases of Paralysis	0	0	0
Cases of Imbecility	8	2	10
Insensible to calls of nature	6	4	10
Refuse food	0	0	0
Dangerous to themselves	5	4	9
Dangerous to others at present	2	1	3
Dangerous to others occasionally	10	3	13
Disposed to destroy Clothing, &c.	8	6	14
In a Noisy Room last week	2	0	2
Under any Day Restraint last week	1	0	1
Under any Night Restraint last week ...	0	0	0
Sick	2	0	2
Under Surgical Treatment	2	0	2

*TABLE XXXI.

Weekly Return of the State of the Patients.

From Dec. 24 to Dec. 31, 1835.	M.	F.	Totals
Number of Patients in the House	41	21	62
First Rank	5	2	7
Second Rank	3	1	4
Third Rank	33	18.	51
Maintained by their Friends	17	7	24
Maintained by the Public	24	14	38
Less than 1 year since the 1st attack ...	7	6	13
More than 1 year since the 1st attack ...	34	15	49
Not expected to recover	31	11	42
Expected to recover	10	10	20
Convalescent	1	2	3
Employed	12	12	24†
Attended Chapel on Sunday	26	13	39
Cases of Idiotcy	1	1	2
Cases of Epilepsy	4	1	5
Cases of Paralysis	0	0	0
Cases of Imbecility	11	1	12
Insensible to calls of nature	7	1	8
Refuse food	0	1	1
Dangerous to themselves	5	5	10
Dangerous to others at present	4	2	6
Dangerous to others occasionally	11	5	16
Disposed to destroy Clothing, &c.	8	4	12
In a Noisy Room	0	0	0
Under any Day Restraint	0	0	0
Under any Night Restraint	0	0	0
Sick	3	0	3
Under Surgical Treatment	2	0	2
Died	0	0	0

Females.—Spinning, Knitting, Needle-work, Cleaning } 11
Wards, &c.
In the Laundry 1

+ Males.—Cleaning Wards, &c. 5
Gardening, Pumping Water, and other out- } 5
door Employment ....
In the Kitchen and Wash-house 2

1836.

*TABLE XXXII.

Number of the Patients Admitted, and of those Discharged from the Books,

From January 1, 1836, to December 31, 1836.

	M.	F.	Tot.
Remained January 1, 1836......................	41	21	62
Admitted in 1836	22	21	43
Re-admitted in 1836	2	8	10
Discharged in 1836	12	18	30
Remaining December 31, 1836	53	32	85

*TABLE XXXIII.

State of the Patients when Discharged from the Books,

From January 1, 1836, to December 31, 1836.

Recovered..	19
Improved	1
Removed during treatment......................................	5
Improper object	0
By order of the Board..	0
Escaped	1
Dead..	4

*TABLE XXXIV.

Causes of the Deaths in 1836.

Apoplexy	1	Dying when admitted......	1
Diseased Heart	1	Gradual Exhaustion	1

*TABLE XXXV.

Weekly Return of the State of the Patients.

From June 27 to July 4, 1836.	M.	F.	Totals
Number of Patients in the House	51	25	76
First Rank	4	1	5
Second Rank	5	3	8
Third Rank	42	21	63
Maintained by their Friends	18	7	25
Maintained by the Public	33	18	51
Less than 1 year since the 1st attack ...	7	5	12
More than 1 year since the 1st attack ...	44	20	64
Not expected to recover	44	18	62
Expected to recover	7	7	14
Convalescent	1	1	2
Employed	18	10	28†
Attended Chapel on Sunday	35	11	46
Cases of Idiotcy	2	0	2
Cases of Epilepsy	5	1	6
Cases of Paralysis	0	1	1
Cases of Imbecility	10	5	15
Insensible to calls of nature	5	4	9
Refuse food	0	1	1
Dangerous to themselves	8	6	14
Dangerous to others at present	8	7	15
Dangerous to others occasionally	17	10	27
Disposed to destroy Clothing, &c.	13	7	20
In a Noisy Room	0	0	0
Under any Day Restraint	0	0	0
Under any Night Restraint	0	0	0
Sick	4	1	5
Under Surgical Treatment	1	0	1
Died	0	0	0

Females.—Spinning, Knitting, Needle-work, Cleaning Wards, &c. ....1 In the Laundry and Kitchen 7 2

† Males.—Cleaning Wards, &c. Gardening, Pumping Water, and other out-door Employment. ....6 9 In the Wash-house, Mangle-house, and Scullery 3

*TABLE XXXVI.

Weekly Return of the State of the Patients.

From Dec. 24 to Dec. 31, 1836.	M.	F.	Totals
Number of Patients in the House	53	32	85
First Rank	4	2	6
Second Rank	4	1	5
Third Rank	45	29	74
Maintained by their Friends	16	7	23
Maintained by the Public	37	25	62
Less than 1 year since the 1st attack ...	2	7	9
From 1 to 2 years since the 1st attack ...	6	1	7
More than 2 years since the 1st attack ...	45	24	69
Less than 1 year since admission	16	14	30
From 1 to 2 years since admission	5	3	8
From 2 to 13 years since admission	21	8	29
Re-admitted cases not included in the above	11	7	18
Not expected to recover	45	25	70
Expected to recover	8	7	15
Convalescent	3	2	5
Employed	23	11	34†
Attended Evening Prayers	17	10	27
Attended Chapel on Sunday	35	10	45
Cases of Idiotcy	2	0	2
Cases of Epilepsy	5	1	6
Cases of Paralysis	0	1	1
Cases of Imbecility	11	4	15
Insensible to calls of nature	7	6	13
Refuse food	0	1	1
Dangerous to themselves	8	11	19
Dangerous to others at present	6	8	14
Dangerous to others occasionally	14	6	20
Disposed to destroy Clothing, &c.	14	11	25
In a Noisy Room	0	0	0
Under any Day Restraint	0	0	0
Under any Night Restraint	0	0	0
Sick	2	1	3
Under Surgical Treatment	5	2	7
Died	0	0	0

Females.—Spinning, Knitting, Needle-work, Cleaning Wards, &c. 2 7 2
In the Laundry ... ...

† Males.—Cleaning Wards, &c. 0
Pumping Water, collecting Snow for the Copper, and other out-door Employment ... 11 3
In the Wash-house, Scullery, &c. ... ...

---

*TABLE XXXVII.

Number of the Patients Admitted, and of those Discharged from the Books,

From January 1, 1837, to December 31, 1837.

	M.	F.	Tot.
Remained January 1, 1837......................	53	32	85
Admitted in 1837	16	17	33
Re-admitted in 1837	8	4	12
Discharged in 1837	27	15	42
Remaining December 31, 1837	50	38	88

*TABLE XXXVIII.

State of the Patients when Discharged from the Books,

From January 1, 1837, to December 31, 1837.

Recovered...	15
Improved	6
Removed during treatment......................	5
Improper object	0
By order of the Board.............................	1
Escaped	0
Dead	15

*TABLE XXXIX.

Causes of the Deaths in 1837.

Consumption ....,	4	Old Age	3
Dropsy.........................	1	Paralysis	1
Epilepsy	1	Typhus Fever	3
Gradual Exhaustion	1	Ulcerated Bowels	1

*TABLE XL.

Weekly Return of the State of the Patients.

From June 26 to July 3, 1837.	M.	F.	Totals
Number of Patients in the House	61	31	92
First Rank	6	2	8
Second Rank	5	1	6
Third Rank	50	28	78
Maintained by their Friends	21	6	27
Maintained by the Public	40	25	65
Less than 1 year since the 1st attack ...	5	5	10
From 1 to 2 years since the 1st attack ...	3	5	8
More than 2 years since the 1st attack ...	53	21	74
Less than 1 year since admission	13	11	24
From 1 to 2 years since admission	11	8	19
From 2 to 14 years since admission	21	6	27
Re-admitted cases not included in the above	16	6	22
Not expected to recover	48	24	72
Expected to recover	13	7	20
Convalescent	2	2	4
Employed	23	14	37†
Attended Evening Prayers	20	14	34
Attended Chapel on Sunday	36	14	50
Cases of Idiotcy	2	0	2
Cases of Epilepsy	4	1	5
Cases of Paralysis	0	1	1
Cases of Imbecility	10	5	15
Insensible to calls of nature	9	6	15
Refuse food	2	0	2
Dangerous to themselves	9	13	22
Dangerous to others at present	7	6	13
Dangerous to others occasionally	18	8	26
Disposed to destroy Clothing, &c.	14	10	24
In a Noisy Room	0	0	0
Under any Day Restraint	0	0	0
Under any Night Restraint	0	0	0
Sick	3	1	4
Under Surgical Treatment	2	0	2
Died	0	0	0

Females.—Spinning 1
Knitting, Needle-work, Cleaning Wards, } 11
&c. .... } 2
In the Laundry and Kitchen ....

† Males.—Cleaning Wards, &c. 10
Gardening, Pumping Water, and other out- } 10
door Employment .... } 2
Repairing the Patients' Clothes ....
In the Wash-house and Scullery ....

*TABLE XLI.

Weekly Return of the State of the Patients.

From Dec. 24 to Dec. 31, 1837.	M.	F.	Totals
Number of Patients in the House	50	38	88
First Rank	5	1	6
Second Rank	2	1	3
Third Rank	43	36	79
Maintained by their Friends	15	7	22
Maintained by the Public	35	31	66
Less than 1 year since the 1st attack ...	3	5	8
From 1 to 2 years since the 1st attack ...	2	7	9
More than 2 years since the 1st attack ...	45	26	71
Less than 1 year since admission	6	12	18
From 1 to 2 years since admission	12	10	22
From 2 to 14 years since admission	20	8	28
Re-admitted cases not included in the above	12	8	20
Not expected to recover	43	28	71
Expected to recover	7	10	17
Convalescent	2	3	5
Employed	25	14	39†
Attended Evening Prayers	23	16	39
Attended Chapel on Sunday	28	17	45
Cases of Idiotcy	2	0	2
Cases of Epilepsy	4	1	5
Cases of Paralysis	1	1	2
Cases of Imbecility	9	6	15
Insensible to calls of nature	5	5	10
Refuse food	2	0	2
Dangerous to themselves	10	14	24
Dangerous to others at present	5	6	11
Dangerous to others occasionally	17	10	27
Disposed to destroy Clothing, &c.	14	13	27
In a Noisy Room	0	0	0
Under any Day Restraint	0	0	0
Under any Night Restraint	0	0	0
Sick	0	2	2
Under Surgical Treatment	1	0	1
Died	0	0	0

Females.—Knitting, Needle-work, Cleaning Wards, &c. } 13
In the Laundry 1

† Males.—Cleaning Wards, &c., Pumping Water, and other out-door Employment 15
In the Wash-house, Mangle-house, and Scullery 7 3

TABLE XLII.

Number of the Patients Admitted, and of those Discharged from the Books,

From January 1, 1838, to December 31, 1838.

	M.	F.	Tot.
Remained January 1, 1838.............	50	38	88
Admitted in 1838	29	28	57
Re-admitted in 1838	6	7	13
Discharged in 1838...................	29	28	57
Remaining December 31, 1838	56	45	101

TABLE XLIII.

State of the Patients when Discharged from the Books,

From January 1, 1838, to December 31, 1838.

Recovered	31
Improved	6
Removed during treatment.....................	8
Improper object	0
By order of the Board...........................	2
Escaped	0
Dead	10

TABLE XLIV.

Causes of the Deaths in 1838.

Apoplexy	2	Dying when admitted......	1
Consumption	1	Erysipelas	1
Diarrhœa...................	1	Gradual Exhaustion	2
Diseased Liver	1	Old Age	1

TABLE XLV.

Weekly Return of the State of the Patients.

From June 25 to July 2, 1838.	M.	F.	Totals
Number of Patients in the House	55	41	96
First Rank	4	1	5
Second Rank	3	3	6
Third Rank	48	37	85
Maintained by their Friends	17	10	27
Maintained by the Public	38	31	69
Less than 1 year since the 1st attack ...	5	3	8
From 1 to 2 years since the 1st attack ...	1	8	9
More than 2 years since the 1st attack ...	49	30	79
Less than 1 year since admission	12	16	28
From 1 to 2 years since admission	5	4	9
From 2 to 14 years since admission	27	13	40
Re-admitted cases not included in the above	11	8	19
Not expected to recover	47	35	82
Expected to recover	8	6	14
Convalescent	1	1	2
Employed	24	16	40†
Attended Evening Prayers	28	17	45
Attended Chapel on Sunday	36	20	56
Cases of Idiotcy	2	0	2
Cases of Epilepsy	6	2	8
Cases of Paralysis	0	1	1
Cases of Imbecility	11	5	16
Insensible to calls of nature	5	5	10
Refuse food	1	0	1
Dangerous to themselves	11	17	28
Dangerous to others at present	7	6	13
Dangerous to others occasionally	18	17	35
Disposed to destroy Clothing, &c.	18	18	36
Under Night Watch	29	23	52
Sick	1	2	3
Under Surgical Treatment	1	0	1
Died	0	1	1

Females.—Knitting, Needle-work, Cleaning Wards, &c. } 14
In the Laundry and Kitchen 2

† Males.—Cleaning Wards, &c. 10
Gardening, Pumping Water, and other out-door Employment } 10
In the Wash-house, Mangle-room, Kitchen, and Scullery } 4

TABLE XLVI.

Weekly Return of the State of the Patients.

From Dec. 24 to Dec. 31, 1838.	M.	F.	Totals
Number of Patients in the House	56	45	101
First Rank	6	3	9
Second Rank	5	2	7
Third Rank	45	40	85
Maintained by their Friends	22	7	29
Maintained by the Public	34	38	72
Less than 1 year since the 1st attack ...	6	3	9
From 1 to 2 years since the 1st attack ...	1	8	9
More than 2 years since the 1st attack ...	49	34	83
Less than 1 year since admission	12	18	30
From 1 to 2 years since admission	1	5	6
From 2 to 15 years since admission	30	13	43
Re-admitted cases not included in the above	13	9	22
Not expected to recover	48	38	86
Expected to recover	8	7	15
Convalescent	1	1	2
Employed	24	19	43†
Attended Evening Prayers	34	24	58
Attended Chapel on Sunday	35	24	59
Cases of Idiotcy	2	0	2
Cases of Epilepsy	7	3	10
Cases of Paralysis	0	1	1
Cases of Imbecility	12	5	17
Insensible to calls of nature	6	7	13
Refuse food	0	0	0
Dangerous to themselves	15	22	37
Dangerous to others at present	6	7	13
Dangerous to others occasionally	18	17	35
Disposed to destroy Clothing, &c.	17	22	39
Under Night Watch	27	23	50
Sick	0	1	1
Under Surgical Treatment	0	2	2
Died	0	0	0

Females,—Knitting, Needle-work, Cleaning Wards, &c. } 15 ◄
In the Laundry and Kitchen ... ... 4 ◄

† Males,—Cleaning Wards, &c. ... 11
Pumping Water, and other out-door Employment ... 9
In the Wash-house, Mangle-room, Kitchen, and Scullery ... 4

TABLE XLVII.

Number of the Patients Admitted, and of those Discharged from the Books,

From April 26, 1820, to December 31, 1838.

	M.	F.	Tot.
Admitted	329	261	590
Re-admitted cases	66	59	125
Discharged	339	275	614
Remained December 31, 1838	56	45	101

TABLE XLVIII.

State of the Patients when Discharged from the Books,

From April 26, 1820, to December 31, 1838.

Recovered	285
Improved	70
Removed during treatment	120
Improper object	1
By order of the Board	15
Escaped	5
Dead	118

TABLE XLIX.

Causes of the Deaths,

From April 26, 1820, to December 31, 1838.

Abscess in the Brain	1	Dropsy	7
Apoplexy	8	Dying when admitted	7
Catalepsy	1	Erysipelas	1
Consumption	5	Epilepsy	9
Diarrhœa	4	Fever	3
Diseased Heart	1	Found dead in bed	2
———— Liver	1	Gradual Exhaustion	28

TABLE XLIX.

(CONTINUED.)

Inflamed Brain	1	Paralysis	2
——— Lungs	2	Psoas Abscess	2
——— Parotid Gland	1	Suicide	7
Locked Jaw	1	Tabes	5
Maniacal Exhaustion	6	Typhus Fever	3
Old Age	7	Ulcerated Bowels	2

Water in the Head 1

TABLE L.

Re-admissions.

Of the 590 Patients Admitted, have been Re-admitted.

73 Patients	....	1 time each	....	73 cases
10	....	2 times each	....	20 ......
2	....	3	....	6 ......
2	....	4	....	8 ......
2	....	5	....	10 ......
1	....	8	....	8 ......
90 Patients				125 cases

TABLE LI.

Of the 285 Patients Discharged as Recovered, have been Re-admitted.

26 Patients	....	1 time each	....	26 cases
4	....	2 times each	....	8 ......
2	....	3	....	6 ......
1	....	4	....	4 ......
1	....	7	....	7 ......
34 Patients				51 cases

Of whom 4 have died, and 3 remain in the Asylum.

TABLE LII.

Recovery as affected by the Duration of the Complaint, before Admission.

Periods of Recovery.	Admitted within 3 months of the 1st attack, 181	Admitted between 3 & 12 mo. of the 1st attack, 112	Admitted between 1 & 2 years of the 1st attack, 37	Admitted, the period of attack being upwards of 2 years, 129	Admitted, having had previous attacks, 231	Admitted, the period of attack not known, 21	Admitted Idiots, 4	Totals.
Discharged within 3 months after admission	68	13	1	2	52	0	0	136
—— between 3 and 6 months after admission	39	8	2	2	30	0	0	81
—— between 6 and 12 months after admission	12	5	4	3	26	0	0	50
—— between 1 and 2 years after admission	1	4	0	1	4	0	0	10
—— between 2 and 3 years after admission	1	0	0	0	0	0	0	1
—— after 3 years	1	0	1	2	3	0	0	7
Totals	122	30	8	10	115	0	0	285

TABLE LIII.

Number of the Patients Admitted in each Year, from April 26, 1820, to December 31, 1838.

1820	1821	1822	1823	1824	1825	1826	1827	1828	1829	1830	1831	1832	1833	1834	1835	1836	1837	1838
15	24	20	22	34	30	35	35	41	41	43	29	37	40	59	42	53	45	70

TABLE LIV.

Number of Patients Admitted in each Month.

Jan.	Feb.	March	April	May	June	July	Aug.	Sep.	Oct.	Nov.	Dec.
48	55	54	61	64	72	65	66	56	53	53	68

TABLE LV.

Ages at the time of Admission.

Betw. 13—20	20—30	30—40	40—50	50—60	60—70	70 & upw.	not known	Total.
35	138	182	151	109	52	19	29	715

TABLE LVI.

Number of Deaths in each Month.

Jan.	Feb.	March	April	May	June	July	Aug.	Sep.	Oct.	Nov.	Dec.
7	9	8	8	12	15	9	14	3	9	13	11

TABLE LVII.

Periods of Decease after Admission.

Between 1—7 days	Days 7—14	Weeks 2—4	Months 1—3	Months 3—6	Months 6—12	Years 1—2	Years 2—3	Years 3—16	Total.
5	8	7	14	13	21	18	10	22	118

TABLE LVIII.

Ages at the time of Decease.

Betw. 13—20	20—30	30—40	40—50	50—60	60—70	70 & upw.	not known	Total.
1	12	24	26	23	13	10	9	118

TABLE LIX.

Employment of the Female Patients,

From January 1, 1838, to December 31, 1838.

Sheets, Pairs of	48	Coarse Socks, Pairs of	5
Towels	72	Fancy Socks & Stockings ... ditto	100
Table Cloths	15		
Beds	24	Garters .... ditto	12
Pillows	24	Pincushion-covers	8
Pillow-cases	60	Petticoats	24
Blanket-cases	2	Flannel Petticoats	27
Straw-cases	6	Shifts	41
Window Blinds	14	Night Gowns	26
Muslin ditto	13	Caps	64
Handkerchiefs	26	Aprons	8
Neck-kerchiefs	12	Flannel Waistcoats	10

From January 1, 1839, to February 14, 1839.

Mattrasses	13	Towels, the Cloth woven from Yarn spun by the Patients	53
Bolsters	96		
Chair Cushions	2		

The Female Patients have repaired the whole of their
own Clothing, the Male Patients' under Clothing, and the
House Linen, with the assistance of a Semptress for two
days weekly.

Note.—The Mattrasses were stuffed by a Semptress.

DIET TABLE.

FIRST AND SECOND RANKS.

Breakfast......Tea or Coffee with Bread and Butter.
Dinner.........Meat with Puddings.
Tea ....With Bread and Butter.
Supper.........Boiled Milk, or Gruel with Currants, Fruit
               Pies occasionally.

THIRD RANK.

MORNING.

Females.........Tea (one pint) with Dry Toast
Males............Gruel (one quart).

DINNERS.

Sunday............Roast Beef.
Monday ....Boiled Mutton.
Tuesday ....Roast Beef.
Wednesday ......Boiled Beef, or Broth, with Hashed Meat.
Thursday.........Boiled Mutton.
Friday............Boiled Beef.
Saturday ....Boiled Beef, or Broth, with Hashed Meat.

EVENING.

Females ....Tea (one pint) with Bread and Butter.
Males ....Boiled Milk (one pint).

Bread and Vegetables, without excess or waste.

FEVER DIET.

For *Dinner*, light Pudding, Broth, Rice, or Gruel.
For *Breakfast* and *Supper*, Tea or Gruel.
For common drink, Toast and Water, or Barley Water.

1838.

Average Consumption of Bread, per head, per day ... 18 oz.
Average Consumption of Meat, per head, per day ... 8½ oz.

F.

TABLE

SHEWING THE PROBABILITIES OF LIFE

IN THE

KINGDOM OF SWEDEN,

ACCORDING TO THE

AVERAGE OF SEVEN DIFFERENT ENUMERATIONS IN

1757, 1760, 1763, 1766, 1769, 1772 & 1775.

Ages.	Numbers Living.	Deaths.	Deaths per Cent.
Between 15—20	58,208	405	0.695
20—30	109,555	1,011	0.922
30—40	98,355	1,200	1.220
40—50	85,177	1,438	1.688
50—60	68,930	1,825	2.647
60—70	48,321	2,348	4.859
70 & upw.	29,154	3,520	12.073

G.

RATE OF MORTALITY AT DIFFERENT AGES

IN THE

LINCOLN ASYLUM,

FROM ENUMERATIONS IN

1832, 1833, 1834, 1835, 1836, 1837 & 1838.

Ages.	Numbers Living.	Deaths.	Deaths per Cent.
Between 15—20	21	1	4.760
20—30	124	5	4.000
30—40	230	17	7.391
40—50	208	12	5.769
50—60	118	15	12,711
60—70	59	6	10.170
70 & upw.	20	6	30.000
not known	6	1	

Classics in Psychiatry

An Arno Press Collection

Feuchtersleben, Ernst [Freiherr] von. **The Principles Of Medical Psychology.** 1847

Georget, [Etienne-Jean]. **De La Folie:** Considérations Sur Cette Maladie. 1820

Haslam, John. **Observations On Madness And Melancholy.** 1809

Hill, Robert Gardiner. **Total Abolition Of Personal Restraint In The Treatment Of The Insane.** 1839

Janet, Pierre [Marie-Felix] and F. Raymond. **Les Obsessions Et La Psychasthénie.** 1903. Two volumes

Janet, Pierre [Marie-Felix]. **Psychological Healing.** 1925. Two volumes

Kempf, Edward J. Psychopathology. 1920

Kraepelin, Emil. **Manic-Depressive Insanity And Paranoia.** 1921

Kraepelin, Emil. **Psychiatrie:** Ein Lehrbuch Für Studirende Und Aerzte. 1896

Laycock, Thomas. **Mind And Brain.** 1860. Two volumes in one

Liébeault, A[mbroise]-A[uguste]. **Le Sommeil Provoqué Et Les États Analogues.** 1889

Mandeville, B[ernard] De. **A Treatise Of The Hypochondriack And Hysterick Passions.** 1711

Morel, B[enedict] A[ugustin]. **Traité Des Degénérescences Physiques, Intellectuelles Et Morales De L'Espèce Humaine.** 1857. Two volumes in one

Morison, Alexander. **The Physiognomy Of Mental Diseases.** 1843

Myerson, Abraham. **The Inheritance Of Mental Diseases.** 1925

Perfect, William. **Annals Of Insanity.** [1808]

Pinel, Ph[ilippe]. **Traité Médico-Philosophique Sur L'Aliénation Mentale.** 1809

Prince, Morton, et al. **Psychotherapeutics.** 1910

Psychiatry In Russia And Spain. 1975

Ray, I[saac]. **A Treatise On The Medical Jurisprudence Of Insanity.** 1871

Semelaigne, René. **Philippe Pinel Et Son Oeuvre Au Point De Vue De La Médecine Mentale.** 1888

Thurnam, John. **Observations And Essays On The Statistics Of Insanity.** 1845

Trotter, Thomas. **A View Of The Nervous Temperament.** 1807

Tuke, D[aniel] Hack, editor. **A Dictionary Of Psychological Medicine.** 1892. Two volumes

Wier, Jean. **Histoires, Disputes Et Discours Des Illusions Et Impostures Des Diables, Des Magiciens Infames, Sorcieres Et Empoisonneurs.** 1885. Two volumes

Winslow, Forbes. **On Obscure Diseases Of The Brain And Disorders Of The Mind.** 1860

Burdett, Henry C. **Hospitals And Asylums Of The World.** 1891-93. Five volumes. 2,740 pages on NMA standard 24x-98 page microfiche only